Aromatherapy

WITH

Essential Oil Diffusers

Aromatherapy

——— WITH ———

Essential Oil Diffusers

FOR EVERYDAY HEALTH & WELLNESS

KARIN PARRAMORE, LAc, CH

For complete cataloguing information, see page 209.

Disclaimer
This book is a general guide only and should never be a substitute for the skill, knowledge and
experience of a qualified medical professional dealing with the facts, circumstances and symptoms
of a particular case.

The medical and health information presented in this book is based on the research, training
and professional experience of the author, and is true and complete to the best of her knowledge.
However, this book is intended only as an informative guide for those wishing to know more about
health and aromatherapy; it is not intended to replace or countermand the advice given by the
reader's personal physician. Because each person and situation is unique, the author and the publisher
urge the reader to check with a qualified health-care professional before using any procedure where
there is a question as to its appropriateness. The author and the publisher are not responsible for
any adverse effects or consequences resulting from the use of the information in this book. It is the
responsibility of the reader to consult a physician or other qualified health-care professional regarding
his or her personal care.

Design and production: Daniella Zanchetta/PageWave Graphics Inc.
Editor: Sue Sumeraj
Proofreader: Kelly Jones
Indexer: Gillian Watts
Illustrations: Kveta/Three in a Box

Cover image: Lavender essential oil © Amy Lv/iStock/Getty Images Plus

Published by Robert Rose Inc.
120 Eglinton Avenue East, Suite 800, Toronto, Ontario, Canada M4P 1E2
Tel: (416) 322-6552 Fax: (416) 322-6936
www.robertrose.ca

Printed and bound in Canada

1 2 3 4 5 6 7 8 9 MI 25 24 23 22 21 20 19 18 17

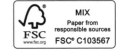

Contents

Introduction

This book is about aromatherapy — specifically, it's about how to diffuse essential oils for improved health and well-being. We hear the term "aromatherapy" used a lot these days, as essential oils become trendier and more people become familiar with them, but what exactly does it mean?

At its most basic level, the meaning of "aromatherapy" is right there in the word itself: the use of aroma in a therapeutic way, to address imbalances in our bodies that can lead to poor health. For a more detailed understanding of how aromatherapy works, read on!

Beware of Misinformation

Unfortunately, like all trends, aromatherapy has generated an awful lot of misinformation, some of which is downright dangerous. Educating yourself about aromatherapy with trustworthy sources (see Resources, page 206), is crucial to avoid jeopardizing your health.

Communicating through Aroma

An aroma, of course, is something that we detect in the air around us using our sense of smell. Plants and animals release scent molecules to communicate with each other, within their own species and across species. We all know that flowers send out their perfume to attract pollinators (and human noses!) so they can get help distributing their pollen. But did you know that plants also use scent as a warning to others of their species? When an infestation of insects starts to decimate a crop, the plants being eaten change their chemical output to deter the pests, changing their flavor so they are less appealing to the insects. These altered chemicals become part of the scent profile the plants release into the air and act to warn the rest of the plants in the crop that they are about to be eaten. When they receive this message, the plants farther afield also change their chemistry to match the message. By the time the insects make their way through the field, the plants become less appealing, and more are spared.

Plants are quite adept at this type of communication, as it is one of their only defenses, being tethered to the ground as they are. But animals also send signals with scent, releasing pheromones to send clear messages to both friends and rivals. We humans have this ability, too, of course. In earlier eras, much of our communication with other humans was carried out by scents we produced in response to emotions. Sexual readiness and interest were signaled by specific pheromones released by attraction, while fear signaled vulnerability to our enemies. But as humanity learned about the dangers of filth in transmitting disease, the natural smells humans create came to be associated with disease transmission, and natural odors were seen as distasteful and something to be avoided. These days, we have, for the most part, lost our ability to communicate pheremonally — at least consciously.

The Dangers of Synthetic Fragrances

Nowadays we are more likely to smell like a synthetic version of flowers, as commercial interests have determined that the use of chemical fragrances is much more financially viable than using natural oils. Unfortunately, our bodies are not capable of processing many of the chemicals we apply to our skin or inhale from outgassing plastics and other synthetic materials. Alarming reports of illness and allergies due to exposure to chemicals are on the rise, especially when it comes to the most vulnerable members of our population: our children.

The most disturbing aspect of synthetic fragrances is their chemical structure. Many are so similar to endogenous (naturally produced) hormones, they have been grouped into the category of "xenoestrogens" — and they function in the body almost exactly like the estrogen we produce naturally. In fact, xenoestrogens often have a greater affinity for hormone receptors and can displace naturally occurring estrogen. Moreover, they stay attached far longer than a natural estrogen molecule would. This can wreak havoc in the endocrine system, which holds the primary responsibility for sending hormonal messages within the body that allow it to function properly.

A Return to Natural Aromas

To stay as healthy as possible, we must strive to avoid endocrine-disrupting, chemically derived synthetic fragrances and return to using scents derived directly from plants. Essential oils are concentrated distillations from various parts of plants with known health benefits. As such, they are instantly recognized by our endocrine and nervous systems, which are able to process essential oil molecules in ways that lead to health improvements rather than health imbalances.

As you become more familiar with these precious plant substances, keep in mind that the production of essential oils is incredibly labor-intensive and requires enormous amounts of

Functional Fragrance

What we perceive as a lovely, often elusive fragrance has a greater function than simply improving our mood (or warning us to avoid spoiled food). Many volatile molecules are released to communicate with other members of a species, for reproductive or safety needs, for example.

Avoiding Synthetics

In addition to the benefits provided by essential oils themselves, the suggestions in this book may help you to avoid some of the synthetic fragrances that are becoming ubiquitous in our modern environment. That benefit alone can lead to greater balance and a healthier life.

raw materials. For example, distilling a pound of eucalyptus oil requires about 50 pounds of leaves; a pound of lavender oil requires about 150 pounds of plant matter; and a pound of rose oil requires about 3,000 pounds of petals! This makes it clear why essential oils are so pricy, but it also helps us understand why 1 drop of oil may be all you need to address an imbalance. With essential oils, less is most definitely more, at least to start.

Keep it Simple

I intentionally kept the oil blends simple, as I have found that blends composed of three essential oils are effective without being overwhelming. As you learn more about how you respond to certain oils, and which ones you prefer, consider my blends to be a jumping-off point for creating your own!

Diffusing Essential Oils

Essential oils can be used for aromatherapy in many different ways: they can be inhaled, applied to the skin, ingested via food or used internally via suppository, douche or enema. This book primarily discusses the use of essential oil diffusion to address health imbalances.

The term "diffusion" means any action that encourages the release of volatile molecules from an essential oil. Just opening a bottle is, in a very basic way, diffusing! Of course, there are many ways to diffuse oils that are a bit more effective than simply opening a bottle. The various options are discussed extensively in "Types of Diffusers" (page 20), and specific instructions on how to best diffuse oils to treat a particular health condition are given with each oil blend in "Improving Your Health with Essential Oils" (page 80).

A great number of health issues can be addressed with this form of aromatherapy, a subject that does not receive as much attention as it ought to. This book attempts to remedy that. The "Improving Your Health with Essential Oils" chapter is arranged by category of health imbalance and includes only those conditions that are well addressed by essential oil diffusion, such as respiratory ailments and mental or emotional imbalances.

In addition, in the "Enhancing Your Environment with Essential Oils" chapter (page 181), I have included suggestions on using essential oil diffusion to resolve issues in your home, work space and car, such as mold in your bathroom or mice in your attic.

I hope you find this book useful, and above all, I hope you enjoy the experience of diffusing essential oils! Best of health to you.

Part 1

....

Essential Oil Diffusion

Scented Plants for Holistic Health: A Short History

Humans have been using plant materials for millennia, for everything from food to shelter, and from clothing to medicine. In these modern times of concrete homes and packaged foods, it is easy to forget how dependent we are on plants, but make no mistake: if plants were to suddenly disappear from the planet, we wouldn't survive for more than a few weeks, at best, and probably mere days.

While we have been distilling essential oils from plants for only a few centuries, we have always found other creative ways to take advantage of plants' volatile compounds. Some of these are explored below.

Further Reading

This chapter merely skims the surface of the information available on the history of scent and scent materials. If you would like to learn more, I have added some suggestions in the Resources (page 206).

Prehistoric Ritual Use

One of the earliest known sites where fragrant plants were used for ritual is in Israel, in a cemetery estimated to be about 13,000 years old. The graves excavated here were found to have been lined with highly fragrant plants, including sage and mint, as well as others that appear to have been chosen for their large or plentiful flowers.

Other factors observed at the site, such as the arrangement of the bodies, confirm that these ancient people were buried in a ritualistic way that would have been enhanced by the use of plants for the scent and color they contributed to the proceedings. Nothing else in the natural world generates the sweet scent associated with flowers, and their fragrance can induce an intoxicated or euphoric state that would enhance the spirituality of a ritual for its participants. Color would also have played a role: after the dull tones of winter, the flowers of spring and summer must have seemed utterly miraculous, a return of life and the vital force.

Let's consider this for a moment. Even in prehistory, flowering plants were recognized as an appropriate symbol for the return of life. The archaeological record seems to indicate that people lined graves with flowers to ensure a successful return to the material world after a journey through the underworld. Being transported back to life by fragrance — what a lovely thought! To this day, the scent of flowers inspires thoughts of youth, hope, renewal and vitality, affecting mood and encouraging hope.

A Reciprocal Arrangement

Sniffing flowers is an act that brings on a sense of calm and relaxation, if not outright euphoria — sensations that tend to encourage repetition. The flowers benefit as well: since they have sent out their fragrance specifically to get help spreading their pollen, when we sniff their flowers, we are helping them to procreate. Is it any wonder that the scent of flowers evokes joy? Or that floral scents have been used for as long as humans have been around to signal sexual readiness and stimulate desire?

Religious Use

All of the major religions, including Christianity, Islam and Judaism, as well as ethical systems such as Buddhism, have long used scent to raise consciousness out of the earthly experience and toward the contemplation of the infinite. In some of the earliest examples, the temples of ancient Mesopotamia are believed to have been built entirely from fragrant wood, like cypress, and Solomon's Temple had doors carved from cedar of Lebanon.

Today, Buddhists in India, China and Japan burn incense at altars, believing the smoke will carry their prayer and devotion. A similar concept is found in Judaism, as burnt offerings. While originally flesh was burned, over time, fragrant plants became more commonly used as offerings.

Christianity

Christianity is inextricably linked with the fragrant resins frankincense and myrrh. They represented two of the three precious gifts carried by the three wise men to the birth of Jesus, and it has been suggested that the third gift, "gold," was actually ambergris, one of the costliest and most precious fragrant substances in existence at the time.

Fragrance, in the form of incense, is still widely used in many Christian sects, especially on high holy days in the Catholic church and the Anglican church, among others. I was recently in Westminster Abbey on a devotional day. The enormous cathedral, walls blackened by centuries of candle smoke and incense, was filled with smoke rising from

The High Cost of Fragrance

Later in his life, Jesus would again come to be associated with fragrance, when Mary Magdalene used anointing oils on his feet: "Mary therefore took a pound of expensive ointment made from pure nard, and anointed the feet of Jesus and wiped his feet with her hair. The house was filled with the fragrance of the perfume." (John 12:3) Judas called Mary Magdalene to task for her extravagance: "Why was this fragrant oil not sold for three hundred denarii and given to the poor?" (John, 12:4–8)

Judas' rebuke is unsurprising when we consider that, in present-day figures, 300 denarii would be somewhere around $30,000!

Fragrant materials have always been extremely expensive, in part because of the incredibly labor-intensive methods required to collect them and in part (especially in ancient times) thanks to the vast distances many of these substances had to travel, as many fragrant plants have quite limited growth zones. A kilogram (about 2 pounds) of jasmine essential oil, one of the more expensive oils, costs around $500 in today's market. To get a kilo of oil, you need over a million jasmine blossoms, all of which must be collected by hand on the first day they bloom, after dawn but before the sun hits them and starts the volatilization process. When you consider these factors, $500 seems like a deal!

Scented Rosaries

A lovely Catholic tradition that continues to this day is the practice of transforming funeral flowers into rosaries. In a religion that places great importance on transition rituals and prayer, this tradition makes sense. The scent of the flowers is captured in the beads, and the scent is released by the warmth of the hand as the petitioner prays.

two gold censers, lazy waves of scent rolling slowly toward the ceiling. It was indeed a transcendent experience.

Anointing oils are used for everything from baptism to exorcism. Holy chrism, the name of the oil used in these rituals, includes resins and balsams in a base of (usually) olive oil. In addition to these fragrant ingredients, the oil contains another key element: the blessing of the bishop. The only time an unsanctified oil may be used is in extremis, if a faithful member of the church is likely to depart before chrism can be found to use in the last rites.

Islam

The founder of Islam, the prophet Mohammed, said, "Every Muslim should have a bath on Friday [the holy day of Islam] and wear his best clothing, and if he has perfume, he should use it." This concept is foundational to the practice of Islam. At every mosque I have visited, in Turkey and Saudi Arabia, but also in European and American mosques, there is a wudu tap: a source of water for the act of wudu, or ritual bathing. Wudu is one of the four obligatory acts of Islam. Many mosques will also be permeated with fragrances to prepare the heart for prayer. I have even seen scent bottles provided, so one can dab oneself before entering the mosque.

The use of perfume in Islamic culture goes back to at least the sixth century. Many of the plants used in scenting agents are native to the regions where Islam first arose, and have been actively cultivated for thousands of years to ensure a plentiful supply. Indonesia is a perfect environment for growing patchouli and ylang ylang; in Pakistan, jasmine and frangipani grow beautifully; and Turkey is home of some of the most exotically delicious rose species.

Due to a ban on the use of alcohol as a base for perfume, most fragrances used by Muslims are authentic attars. These substances are actually quite medicinal, as they are made in the ancient and authentic manner: solely with plant material and healing oils. One scent, called oud, is purported to have almost magical powers of transformation and is widely used in many Islamic countries in both incense and perfumery. Oud is distilled from agarwood, but only after it has been attacked by a mold that transforms the wood from a pale odorless substance to a dark, richly scented material.

Scent Memories

I grew up in Saudi Arabia, the original home of Mohammed and the birthplace of Islam. This greatly influenced my love of scent. One of my earliest memories is walking through the souk, surrounded by enormous mounds of frankincense and myrrh resin "tears," their heady scent released into the air by the intense heat.

My father was something of a diplomat, and one day, our entire family was invited to the home of the oil minister, Sheikh Yamani. We drove through the winding hills of Taif before arriving at his palatial estate. As we entered his home, we were offered a censer of burning resin to freshen us after our drive. Because most people in Saudi Arabia wear clothing that is open from the bottom, we were instructed to stand over the rising smoke for a second or two. It is a memory I cherish.

Social and Medicinal Use

Of course, fragrance is not limited to religious or ritual use. To this day, fragrance is used in all aspects of social interaction, and even conventional medicine uses scent in hospitals for its calming influence. These practices are not new; we merely follow in a long tradition of using plants and fragrance wherever possible!

Ancient Egypt

In Ancient Egypt, scent was understood to be secretions from the sun god, Ra. Fragrance was used in every aspect of everyday life, with no great distinction being made between ritual, medical and social uses. The same blend of fragrant herbs and oils might be used as protection against evil spirits and to treat digestive complaints.

One formula in particular was used for a great variety of complaints. Called *kap-t* in Egyptian, its name was later changed to the Greek *kyphi*. While the Egyptians used many different blends, *kyphi* is probably the most famous, as several different variations on the formula were recorded. *Kyphi* always contained many different fragrant ingredients, including cassia, cinnamon, mastic, mint, juniper berries, cardamom and spikenard. Many of these highly aromatic plant parts are also strongly antimicrobial and make very effective medicinals.

A fascinating (and to modern sensibilities, slightly bizarre) Egyptian practice, described in hieroglyphics and shown in pictographs, was the use of bitcones. A bitcone was a creation shaped from waxes that had been impregnated with fragrant plant material. These cones were worn on the head and slowly melted in the heat of the blazing Nile Valley, gradually dripping fragrant oils over the head and body.

Bitcones are primarily shown on the heads of courtesans, so it may be that they were used to stimulate sexual desire, but it is more likely that they were used to cover the smell of body odor. The lubrication provided would also have helped combat the drying effects of intense sun exposure, and healing oils may have helped with skin conditions.

Ancient Rome

The Ancient Romans were noted for their oil treatments, especially in conjunction with their bath houses, which they built in nearly every land they conquered. Introducing public baths to the so-called barbaric lands may have been the Romans' greatest contribution to the development of Western society (after roads, perhaps).

Typically, the Romans used olive oil to clean grime off their skin. The oil would be generously rubbed into the skin, then scraped off with a strigil (a flat wooden paddle). Only then would they soak in the waters of the bath. After the soak, it was common to have a massage, using more olive oil, often scented with fragrant plants.

From the decadent last years of the Roman Empire comes a story of perhaps the most ostentatious use of scenting materials ever recorded. The Emperor Nero was a mad fan of roses and regularly used both rose petals and rose water to scent his private parties (to be fair, he also decreed that it should be used in public spaces, though less extravagantly). He had special pipes made of silver installed in his residence for the sole purpose of spritzing rose water over his guests. One alarming story claims that he once dropped so many rose petals on his guests, he actually suffocated one of them. Sir Lawrence Alma-Tadema's painting *The Roses of Heliogabalus* (1888) depicts a similar scene and gives some idea of the floral excesses of Nero.

China

The Ancient Chinese were deeply connected to the natural world around them. From medicine to art, nature was the inspiration for nearly every aspect of Chinese life. Confucius used the orchid's fragrance as a symbol of purity, reflecting the virtues that all people should strive to achieve: "If you are in the company of good people, it is like entering a room full of orchids. After a while, you become soaked in the fragrance and you don't even notice it. If you are in the company of bad people, it is like going into a room that smells of fish. After a while, you don't notice the fishy smell as you have been immersed in it."

Scent was a large part of everyday life in Ancient China. Fans, carried by most members of the upper class, were often made from sandalwood so that every time the fan was flicked open the scent would release into the air. Calligraphy, one of the four noble arts of Tang dynasty China, was created using scented inks on paper embedded with fragrant plant material. Statues of the Buddha carved from fragrant camphor wood acted to both scent the room and deter pests.

Empress Dowager Cixi — the Dragon Empress — lived a classic rags-to-riches story. She started her adult life as a concubine but rapidly rose in influence until she was the ruling power. She was also known for being completely besotted with fragrance, regularly using oils created from a variety of different flowers, such as rose and honeysuckle. The fact that this penchant was recorded in official documents is testament to the degree of her obsession.

As It Was, So It Shall Be

Many of the essential oils used in this book have the same indications as those described for the herbs in the *Shennong Ben Cao Jing*. For example, chamomile was then, and is now, seen as beneficial for headache.

Prescribing Herbs by "Nature"

When I was a student of Chinese medicine, I was delighted to learn that some herbs are prescribed according to their "nature," a term that encompasses many aspects of the medicinal qualities the herb offers. The fragrance, or pungency, of certain herbs is understood to have very specific effects in the body.

This idea is not exclusive to Chinese medicine, of course, but having studied Western herbal concepts for 35 years, I can say with confidence that the Chinese delineation of "nature" is far more detailed and rich. Their model is foundational to some of the concepts in this book and, along with the system devised by Ibn Sina (see page 16), contributed greatly to the natures described in "64 Useful Essential Oils" (pages 43–74).

The empress was not alone in her love of fragrance: Chinese literature describes the distillation of nectars and flowers, like Confucius' favored lotus, as well as chrysanthemum and lily, to wear as scents.

An interesting reference for the medicinal use of plants in Ancient China is *The Classic of Mountains and Seas*, written over the span of thousands of years (the "final" version we know today is from the Han dynasty). While this book is primarily about mythology, the authors describe many fragrant plants commonly used for healing, including the use of plants in poultices for skin conditions.

Shennong Ben Cao Jing (*The Divine Farmer's Materia Medica Classic*), written over 1,500 years ago, covers 365 herbs and other medicinal substances. In some cases, the author refers directly to the scent of an herb and its effects in (or on) the body — there are over 2,000 references to herbs from the perspective of the scent they produce.

Persia

Many of the medicinals from fragrant plants that made their way to Europe arrived via Islam, especially during the Middle Ages. Islam has traditionally encouraged scholarship and learning, and was responsible for bringing much of the classical (Greek and Roman) knowledge to the West at a time when Europe was struggling to escape (in many cases) barbaric conditions and wave after wave of disease, like the bubonic plague.

The works of the Persian philosopher Ibn Sina (or Avicenna, as he came to be called in the West) preserved the knowledge of classical physicians like Galen and extensively expanded on an incredibly wide variety of subjects. When they reached Europe, Ibn Sina's books foundationally reshaped the West's understanding of the natural sciences, philosophy, poetry, astronomy, psychology, chemistry and, of course, medicine.

His great medical treatise, *The Canon of Medicine*, was used for centuries as the foundational text on the subject. His chapter headings cover the gamut — drugs, cosmetics, anatomy, organ function and disease — and reflect the lack of distinct disciplines in a time when knowledge was more universally understood. His section on fragrant plant material uses a system of temperatures, natures and degrees very similar to the system being used at the time (and to this day) in China to classify medicinal substances.

Did You Know?

Ibn Sina is also credited with the creation of the still — without which we would not have essential oils!

Medieval Europe

That is not to say there was no herbal tradition in Europe before Ibn Sina. The Saxon *Leech Book of Bald* dates from around 900 AD, and the fact that an intact copy survives today suggests the information was widely circulated at the time. Interestingly, the book describes the use of vapors for healing, as well as the use of herbal baths — two of the main concepts addressed in this book, as they are still incredibly effective treatments. The Saxon book's thorough materia medica details the particular qualities associated with the plants native to the region.

The 12th-century German abbess and mystic Hildegard von Bingen believed that "the smell of the bud of the lily and the smell of the flowers themselves cheer a person's heart and make a person's thinking right." In addition to the lily's emotional benefits, its leaves were used to treat the skin, especially against poisons and burns, and its root was used in topical treatments to keep the skin looking youthful. These indications could as easily have come from a modern-day text on herbal medicine or aromatherapy!

It has been suggested that, during the repeated outbreaks of the Black Death, the perfumers of the European continent survived in much greater numbers than other populations thanks to the antimicrobial volatile compounds to which they were regularly exposed. Plague doctors took to stuffing beak-like masks with fragrant materials in the belief that the beneficial exudations would offset the pestilential vapors. The story of Dr. Nathaniel Hodges, a doctor who recorded the experience of seeing patients during the Great Plague, is a fascinating account:

> To ward off the infection, he brought along chafing dishes with coals. He ignited them and placed them at the entryway, before the windows, and under the beds if there was enough space. Quicklime, thrown onto the coals along with various spices and herbs, produced a penetrating steam "to destroy the efficacy of the pestilential miasmata."

Despite the fact that only the wealthiest strata of medieval society could afford costly perfumes and fragrant medicinals, every household, from the royal palaces to the poorest serf's hut, would have covered the floors with strewing herbs.

Did You Know?

Hildegard von Bingen was a fascinating person and a polymath. In addition to her medical works, she was a prodigious writer on many topics and a frequent political commentator. She painted beautiful works depicting her visions and wrote a great deal of music, much of which is still being performed to this day.

Strewing Hops

Hops were also used as strewing herbs — somewhat oddly, as hops tend to have a sedative effect. Perhaps the use of this plant was limited to the pubs and drinking houses, where they were first used to brew the ales!

Ostensibly used to soak up the effluvia of daily living, like urine, spit and food droppings, the plants inevitably included fragrant herbs, chosen in part to help cover the stench of unwashed bodies living in close quarters. If a plant releases scent when crushed, it is likely to have medicinal properties, so as the inhabitants went about the activities of daily living, repeatedly stepping on these plants, they were in effect treating their houses and themselves to the benefits of the volatile molecules released.

One of the more commonly used herbs was thyme, noted for its ability to discourage household pests. Thyme grows all over the world in one variety or another and was readily accessible. Sweet marjoram, winter savory and lavender — all of which have highly antimicrobial volatile secretions — were also frequently strewn, as were peppermint and pennyroyal, presumably to add a fresh minty fragrance to the air, although these plants are also antimicrobial.

The same fragrant plants used for strewing were often grown right by the door, so that every time someone entered the house they would brush against them and release the volatile molecules into the air, helping to banish "pestilential vapors."

Victorian Era

By the Victorian era, strewing herbs were no longer used, as the housing conditions had improved (at least for the upper and middle classes; the poor were still suffering in appallingly squalid conditions). Instead, scenting agents became a bit more personal. Women carried small nosegays to sniff whenever encountering distasteful smells, and it was very common to scent the material from which clothing was made. Gloves, in particular, were often scented (see sidebar).

Sweet Gloves

The art of making "sweet gloves," as they were called in the Victorian era, involved massaging the leather with oils or other fats, often lard, scented with a variety of fragrant plants, such as clove, rose, violet, neroli and angelica. Scenting agents from animals, like ambergris and musk, were also used.

The shawls so ubiquitous to Victorian dress came mainly from India. Because these shawls were made from silk and cashmere, entire shipments could be destroyed by insect infestations before reaching the shops in Europe. To combat this, the weavers packed the shawls with packets of patchouli leaves, whose scent is known to drive away pests. In this way, the scent of patchouli became well-known in England, and the sale of patchouli oil skyrocketed.

Native America

This short history would not be complete without mention of Native American sweat lodges. Although thought to be primarily ceremonial, sweat lodges have, in fact, always been a place where deep healing occurs on all levels: mental, emotional, spiritual and physical. The intense heat encourages the body to clear impurities through the skin while also challenging the participants to face their limits and preconceptions as they struggle to deal with air so hot it can hurt to breathe.

Several herbs are traditionally used in the lodge. Sage is often used at the beginning and end of the ritual, and cedar needles may be used directly on the fire during the ceremony itself. Sage is cleansing on every level, while cedar offers support, both spiritual and emotional. Cedar can also strengthen the will, further helping the participants endure the challenges that arise from the experience.

Did You Know?

Sweat lodges have been a part of Native American spiritual practice for a very long time, and many nations still use them today. The lodges are traditionally made from willow withies and animal skins, but many modern lodges use alternative materials, such as canvas.

Keep on Learning!

There is, of course, so much more that could be added to this brief history — entire continents have been left out. In Australia, for example, the indigenous people have a rich herbal history, and many of the plants whose oils are featured in this book (tea tree, eucalyptus) are native to Australia. Still, I hope this introduction will pique your interest! I encourage you to learn as much as you can about essential oils, on every level, if you plan to use them regularly.

Types of Diffusers

Throughout history, people have been enormously creative when it comes to finding ways to add scent to themselves and their environment. While it is fascinating to look back on the pomades and salves, oils and unguents that were so popular for so long, in modern times, people seem to prefer aromas to linger in the air and have created a wide variety of ways to get scent molecules to hover around them, including many types of essential oil diffusers.

Hang 'Em High

If you plan to hang danglers in an area where children might see them, be sure to hang them high enough that they cannot reach them. While a great deal of the essential oil molecules will volatilize away, there will always be some residual oil on the pad that might be irritating to kids' skin and eyes if they happen to touch the dangler.

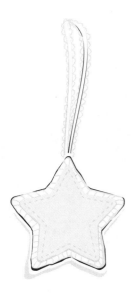

Passive Diffusers

A passive diffuser is any receptacle that holds essential oils and allows the scent of the oils to dissipate into the air through their natural volatility. In most cases, passive diffusers are low-tech and very inexpensive, whether store-bought or DIY.

Absorbent Felt Danglers

Felt danglers are a great way to discreetly diffuse scent wherever you like. The first image that popped into your head when you read the phrase "absorbent felt danglers" was likely the pine tree–shaped pads so commonly seen hanging from car rear-view mirrors. But, although the concept is basically the same, those car danglers tend to be impregnated with synthetic oils that, far from helping, often lead to imbalances, especially in chemically sensitive individuals.

You can make your own felt danglers to hang in your home and your car, using authentic essential oils — and the shape of the felt pad can be whatever you like! Felt danglers can be really fun and can customize the way you diffuse scent. You can purchase stiff, absorbent, feltlike paper from supply companies (see Resources, page 207) or you can use actual wool felt. Simply cut out the desired shape (using a template can help with complicated designs) and punch a hole in the top for the string. Be sure to place the dangler on a horizontal surface before adding drops of essential oils, so they stay in place, and let them absorb into the felt before hanging the dangler.

As long as the scent profile remains the same, you can reuse felt danglers many times. I have found that they can be used for about 3 months before they need to be replaced. The residual oil will eventually oxidize, and oxidized oils are no longer therapeutic. In fact, they can cause sensitivities in a small percentage of the population. If you start noticing that the felt pad smells "off" (which will mean something different depending upon the oils you used), toss your dangler and make another.

Terra Cotta Discs

Terra cotta discs may be my favorite way to passively diffuse scent. These small discs are usually glazed on one side and unglazed on the other. They can be placed glazed side down on any surface, but preferably in a warm spot, like a sunny windowsill. The glazed side will protect the surface the disc rests on, so they can be used in many different areas. If you are at all worried about staining the surface underneath, you can place the disc on a saucer first. (I have seen terra cotta discs that are entirely unglazed; if you choose to use this type, it is important to protect your surface first, as the oils may seep through the disc.)

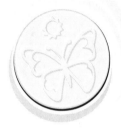

Because the unglazed side of the terra cotta is very porous, it easily holds a drop or two of an essential oil or blend. The warmth of the surroundings then slowly diffuses the scent into the air over time. I have found that the discs will spontaneously release little wafts of scent even after I think all of the essential oil is used up — a sweet surprise!

Cotton Pads and Balls

These are a quick and easy way to diffuse essential oils whenever and wherever they are needed. The cotton facial pads used for removing makeup make fantastic reservoirs for essential oils, as they lay flat, whereas cotton balls can roll off a surface. Another advantage is that the pads can be folded in half to contain the oils, which will make them last longer. If you like to diffuse many different scents throughout the day, or to diffuse scents in different areas of your house or work space, consider buying a packet of these cotton rounds for convenience.

Cotton balls can be very handy for sticking into corners and other small spaces. For example, if you want to diffuse essential oils to help you sleep, add a drop of one of the sleep aid blends (pages 106–107) to a cotton ball and tuck it into the corner of your pillowcase. Make sure to place it strategically so that it will not be near your eyes when your head is on the pillow. It is a good idea to use an old pillowcase, as the oils may stain the cloth.

In fact, when using cotton pads or balls, it is always important to protect the surfaces they are placed on, as there is nothing stopping the oil from seeping through the cotton

Car Scents

You can also use a terra cotta disc to diffuse scent in the car. A non-slip pad, like the ones found in auto parts stores to hold sunglasses on the dashboard, may help to hold it in place. Be sure to remove the disk from the sun after use, especially in hot areas; the oils that remain on the disc will rapidly oxidize if it is left to bake in the sun.

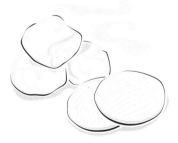

Some aromatherapists use cotton buds to diffuse essential oils, adding a drop of a single oil or blend to the cotton on one end of the bud and placing the other end in a supporting device, such as a small glass or a piece of clay.

and staining the underlying area. You can place a small plastic bag under the pad or ball, and then use it to store the ball or pad when it's not in use. Keep in mind that these are really meant for single or short-term use, however; it's better to use a new one each time!

Avoid touching sensitive tissues, like your eyes, after preparing a cotton pad or ball — it's best to wash your hands immediately, just in case — and, of course, dispose of the cotton properly when you're done with it.

DIY Net Bags

Add a few drops of essential oil to a cotton ball or pad — or a small piece of felt, for that matter — and place it in a small net bag. (I have been known to cut the toes out of pantyhose and use the toes for this purpose.) Using cedarwood essential oil and hanging the net bag in the closet can help drive away moths without having to rely on mothballs. Or use lemon essential oil and hang the bag in the cabinet under the sink to drive out musty odors. Attics, basements and bathrooms all benefit from the cleansing and clearing scent of essential oils diffused in this way. While similar devices are available commercially, the DIY version works just as well!

Reed Diffusers

You may have seen reed diffusers for sale in stores. Unfortunately, they usually come with a really strong synthetic fragrance blend. But these sets can be adapted for use with essential oils instead: simply add the blend you would like to use to a small amount of water, pour the mixture into the vase and insert the reeds. Most oils are hydrophobic, so they will migrate away from the water and into the reeds fairly quickly. Be sure to change the water frequently.

Another fun do-it-yourself option is to dry lavender or other fragrant plant stems, then use them in place of reeds in any small vase you have on hand. The dry stems will quickly absorb the oils and wick them up and out into the air. I have done this with melissa and rosemary stems with great success!

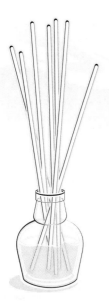

Heat-Activated Diffusers

This type of diffuser is fantastic for creating a mood. In fact, I recommend them mainly for times when the goal is to create an atmosphere that can offset mental distress, calm the mind or enable one to ignore distractions. Because heat changes the chemical structure of essential oils, which can affect their balancing benefits, this type of diffuser is not the best choice for therapeutic use. But if the idea is to add a note to the air, suggest a mood or offset a disagreeable odor, a heat-activated diffuser may be just the thing.

Heating Things Up
Candle-heated diffusers may be particularly helpful in the bedroom, when using a blend to increase libido (see page 99), as the soft glow of the candle may enhance the effects of the oils.

Candle-Heated Diffusers

These popular diffusers are widely available in stores. They typically have a small chamber that holds a candle, with a shallow receptacle above for essential oils. Water is usually added to the receptacle first, in essence creating a kind of mini-steamer that releases moisture and scent, although in truth, the heat from the candle is rarely enough to create steam.

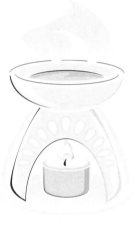

Candle-heated diffusers are often very decorative, with designs ranging from rustic and charming to sleek and modern, and from funky and psychedelic to understated and classic.

Scented Wax Warmers

These work much like candle-heated diffusers but use paraffin wax instead of water as the base for the oils. The wax is heated by either a candle or an electric bulb in the chamber below the wax receptacle, so they emit light as well as scent.

The wax is sold commercially with names like wax melts, wax cookies or wax tarts, but it is best to avoid using synthetic paraffin, if possible, and it is easy to make your own scented wax forms. Simply melt soy, palm or bee's wax in a dedicated pot (or in a glass jar in a bain-marie), then pour the melted wax into a mold, such as a muffin pan lined with paper cupcake liners. Before the wax hardens, add a few drops of a single oil or a prepared blend and swirl it in with a toothpick or bamboo skewer.

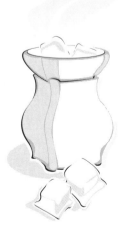

Keep in mind that melted wax can be difficult to remove from the wax warmer's receptacle, so changing scent profiles may be problematic.

Burning Plants

Humans have burned plants to diffuse scent for thousands of years. The practice is especially common in religious or spiritual settings, where the plants were often chosen for their ability to affect people's mental or emotional state, making them more receptive to messages or signs from the gods. For more on this practice, see the box on page 197.

Stovetop Diffusers

A heatproof dish on a woodstove (or a heater) is a really easy way to scent your space, provided the effect is not intended to be medicinal. It is great in winter to help keep the house from smelling musty or stale. All that is required is a dish or bowl that can tolerate high temperatures, water and a drop or two of essential oil. Be careful, though! The water will quickly evaporate, so be sure to keep a close eye on it and refill it as needed.

It should go without saying that the dish will be very hot, so use caution when removing it from the stove or heater.

Another option is to use a saucepan or kettle of water on a gas or electric stovetop. The downside is that the stove must be kept on, which is a waste of energy if you're not cooking; on the other hand, if you *are* cooking, the scent of your oils may be lost in the cooking smells. When I use this method, I place a pan with an inch of water on a burner I just finished using, to take advantage of the remaining radiant heat. That way, there is no wasted energy and the sweet smell from the pan will help clear cooking odors. Plus, you won't need to monitor it, as the burner is off.

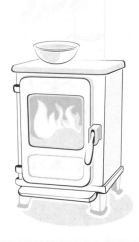

Add Plant Solids

The diffused scent emanating from your stove will last longer if you also add plant material, like cinnamon sticks or juniper berries, to the mix.

Heat-and-Water-Activated Diffusers

Many essential oils are hydrophobic (water-fearing), meaning they will actively attempt to escape a watery environment. Heat compounds this effect, as it contributes to the molecular activity known as volatility. Combining essential oils with heat and water is a fantastic way to ensure their volatilization.

Baths

Bathing is beneficial in so many ways, and even more so when you add essential oils to the water, either on their own or in bath salts. Although we typically think of a full-body bath when we hear the word, there are other types of baths — sitz baths and foot baths — that have specific therapeutic uses, discussed below.

For all baths, you should use warm, not hot, water. The best temperature for a bath is around 100°F (38°C). Water even slightly hotter can impair blood flow, especially for the elderly. For comparison, hot tap water is typically about 114°F (42°C).

First Warm, Then Cool

As difficult as it may be, it is important to follow any warm bath with cool water, whether it's a short rinse under the shower or a brief scrub with a cool washcloth. Here's why: warm water is vasodilating, meaning it lowers blood pressure, but only if the bath is short. If you have ever felt dizzy after a hot bath, it's because blood takes longer to get to your head, thanks to the effects of prolonged vasodilation. A cool water finish promotes vasoconstriction and healthy blood flow.

Full-Body Baths

The full immersion of your body into warm water almost immediately reduces stress on all levels: the buoyancy releases your body from the burden of weight-bearing; the warmth eases soreness and tension; and the reclined position signals your body that it's time to relax. A full-body bath is an excellent way to relax at the end of the day, especially if stress or tension is disrupting your sleep. It is also highly recommended for the first few days when you are starting a new workout routine — ouch!

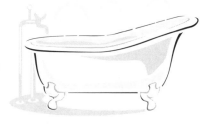

Sitz Baths

The sitz bath, a shallow bath designed for sitting, is used to treat conditions from the hips down. It is often used during and after childbirth, and helps to relieve the pain of hemorrhoids, among other things.

While tubs made specifically for sitz baths are available, any large basin can be used. Be sure to place your sitz bath in the bathtub before use, as much of the water will be displaced by your body when you sit down.

Did You Know?

The word "sitz" comes from the German *sitzen*, meaning "to sit."

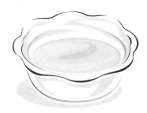

Foot Baths

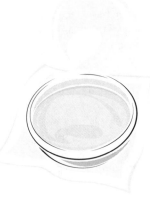

While we generally use a foot bath to treat the feet, in some cases, soaking the feet actually benefits another part of the body. For example, a foot bath may help relieve a headache. Immersing your feet in warm water with a warming oil like ginger encourages vasodilation (the opening of blood vessels), which can help draw congestion out of your head. In addition, essential oils volatilize up from the foot bath, boosting the healing process via the olfactory system as you inhale them.

Because diffusion takes place a bit farther from the nose with a foot bath than with many other diffusion methods, strong oils can be used; in the moment it takes the volatile molecules to rise from the bath to your head, their impact is softened. Thyme essential oil, for instance, is beneficial for respiratory infections but has a very strong scent that is irritating to some people. Using it in a foot bath, to allow it to disperse somewhat before it hits the nose, moderates the irritation.

Healing Help

To enhance the effectiveness of a foot bath for dealing with headaches, add a drop of peppermint essential oil to cool water and use it as a compress on the back of your neck. While the warm foot bath is encouraging vasodilation, the cool compress has the opposite effect: vasoconstriction (the narrowing of blood vessels). Vasoconstriction near your head and vasodilation at your feet creates a pumping action that can really help reduce pressure in your head.

Using Oils in the Bath

Better Incorporation

Adding the oils to an emulsifying agent, such as lecithin, can help to incorporate them into the water.

Adding a drop or two of an essential oil or blend to a bath is a very effective means of diffusion, especially when it comes to strongly scented oils, like lavender or orange.

When taking a full-body bath, be sure to add the oil or blend *after* you get in the tub, because hydrophobic essential oils will immediately disperse over the surface of the water as they try to "flee" it. Once they are spread out, these oils will more readily volatilize away. If you are already in the tub, you will have greater exposure time to the effects of the oils.

Another reason it is important to add oils when you're already in the bath is that there are some less hydrophobic oils that will pool instead of dispersing. If a caustic oil like cinnamon pools in the tub and you happen to sit in this pool, it can be extremely uncomfortable — the tissues that hit the water first as you sit are some of the most sensitive tissues we have.

For sitz baths, on the other hand, you want to add the oils *before* you sit down in the basin. Whatever painful condition is inspiring you to use a sitz bath, it will benefit from direct contact with the diluted essential oils once they have dispersed over the surface of the water.

Using Bath Salts

If you want the scent of the essential oils to last longer in your full-body bath or foot bath, add the oils to salt first. You can use either sodium chloride (such as kosher salt or coarse sea salt) or magnesium sulfate, more commonly known as Epsom salts. Essential oils benefit from the partnership with salt and the warm water of a bath in two ways: the salt slows the diffusion of the volatile molecules, while the warm water helps disperse the molecules across the contained area provided by the tub.

If you are soaking in the tub to reduce pain, such as muscle aches, arthritis or menstrual cramps, Epsom salts are a better choice than sodium chloride, as they are widely believed to help decrease pain and relax muscles. You can increase their benefit by adding essential oils with the same pain-relieving focus, like peppermint or eucalyptus.

To make bath salts, simply add a drop of your favorite single oil or blend to a scant handful of salt in a glass or cup, stir or shake the contents gently, then toss the salts into the tub once you are settled comfortably in it. For the reasons discussed under "Using Oils in the Bath," be sure to add the oil-enhanced salts *after* you get in the tub.

Bath Salt Benefits

Bath salts change the mineral content of the water, increase buoyancy and may help to soften the skin. You can enhance their benefits by adding other ingredients, such as fresh herbs or goat's milk, to your bath. (It is said Cleopatra bathed in donkey's milk!)

Warm Steams

Any time you add essential oils to warm (not hot!) steaming water, you are diffusing them, and you will benefit from the effects. Steam can be created in various ways, both routine and creative, and although commercial steamers and humidifiers are readily available and relatively affordable, there are also plenty of low-cost ways to create steam.

Showers

When you add essential oils to a sponge or washcloth, to unscented liquid or bar soap, to shampoo or conditioner, or to the unglazed grout between your shower tiles, you are, in effect, turning your shower into a giant steamer. The warm, moist air helps deliver the oil molecules to your skin, where they easily cross into your bloodstream. In addition, you inhale a large proportion of the volatile compounds, receiving their benefits through the olfactory system as well.

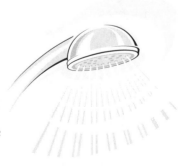

Did You Know?

There is no better treatment than shower diffusion for respiratory imbalances that benefit from warm steam — but not all do, so be careful!

There are many opportunities for using essential oils in the shower: add them to your routine and start the day right every morning with the Wake Up! blend (page 95); reduce aches and pains by using an oil that helps release tension, such as peppermint or lavender; relieve respiratory issues by breathing in warm, fragrant steam to help open your airways; or soothe rashes and breakouts and improve your skin tone with one of the many skin treatment blends in the "Skin Health" section (pages 146–162).

Creative Steaming

Get creative with your steam diffusion techniques! I have a friend who uses lavender hydrosol in her iron to lightly infuse her clothes with the scent. You could do something similar with a curling or straightening iron: before styling, simply spritz your hair lightly with a hydrosol or an essential oil blend in water. Shake well before spritzing!

When you're brainstorming new and clever ways to use steam, do keep in mind that some essential oils are caustic and may damage plastic. Be careful about using them in plastic devices, and try to keep them off the plastic parts of things like irons and hair dryers.

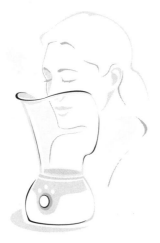

Facial Steamers

These incredibly handy commercial devices direct steam just where you want it, improving the experience by focusing the treatment. Diffusing oils exactly where they are needed is smart and economical, whether you are treating your facial skin, your mouth, your nose or your respiratory system in general. If you find yourself regularly dealing with health imbalances in one or more of these areas, it might be worth considering purchasing a facial steamer.

If face-directed steam is more of an occasional need, however, it is quite easy to create your own facial steamer: all you need is a towel and a bowl of very warm water. Avoid hot water, which could create potentially damaging steam. Generally speaking, one drop of a single oil or blend in a medium mixing bowl is enough, no matter what health issue you are addressing.

Be sure to keep your eyes closed when using a facial steamer, especially if using strong or harsh oils, like peppermint or thyme. The tender tissues of the eyes are easily irritated by both the steam and the oils. (Having said that, I have used hydrosols in my facial steamer specifically to treat irritated eyes. Green myrtle, blue chamomile or lavender hydrosol can all ease painful or itchy eyes.)

Controlling Variables

One advantage of store-bought facial steamers is that they automatically regulate variables such as temperature that may be more difficult to control with a homemade version.

Steaming Chairs

If hemorrhoids or vaginal imbalances are a recurring problem, you may want to invest in a steaming chair or stool. These devices look a bit like a toilet seat on top, but have a shelf underneath that holds a steam basin. Warm water and essential oils are added to the basin, creating steam that is directed exactly where it is needed. The warm, moist treatment is soothing and can help decrease inflammation and lessen pain while reducing microbial loads.

If you don't have a steaming chair, try sitting on a slatted stool over a steam bowl. These stools are commercially available for use in the bathroom or spa.

To use a steaming chair, add a few drops of a single oil or blend to the water in the steaming bowl and sit over it for at least 15 minutes. Contain the steam by wrapping a large towel or sheet over your lap and around the chair. This can be repeated up to three times a day for up to a month. If no benefits are seen, discontinue use.

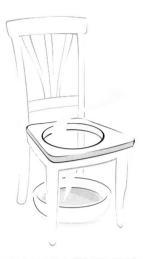

Did You Know?

Steaming chairs have a long history of use with plant material and are easily adapted to use with essential oils.

DIY Steaming Chair

A steaming chair is quite easy to make at home. Find an old wooden chair at a used furniture store, drill a small hole in the seat so you can insert a jigsaw, then cut a larger hole in the center of the seat. Be sure not to cut away so much that you can no longer sit comfortably! Take a look at a toilet seat first for an idea of how much edge to leave. Once the hole is cut, place a bowl of very warm water under the chair, add a drop of your chosen oil or blend, and sit down. Contain the steam by wrapping a sheet or a large towel around the chair and over your lap.

Another option is to securely attach a toilet seat to a 5-gallon (20 L) bucket. Place the basin in the bucket and take a seat!

Humidifiers

If you need a humidifier in your home anyway, it can be a good way to diffuse essential oils into a room. In fact, some humidifiers come with a reservoir specifically designed to hold essential oils, though these are somewhat self-limiting as the reservoir is small and can hold only a few drops.

Is your house dry? Add moisturizing oils like chamomile or fir. If dry conditions are making it difficult to sleep, add orange or spikenard. If you have an active respiratory imbalance, try rosemary or pine.

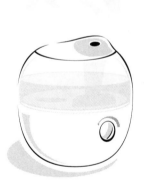

Heal Dry Skin

Humidifiers really help with dry, cracked skin, and you can enhance this benefit by adding an essential oil that improves blood flow, such as carrot seed.

Electric Diffusers

Frankly, I am not a big fan of electric diffusers, whether they are fan-driven or use a heating element, because they diffuse most essential oils too quickly. Their main advantage is that they are usually quite affordable, though they also tend to wear out pretty fast. However, they can be useful for diffusing thicker, more viscous oils that other types of diffusers cannot handle.

Fan Diffusers

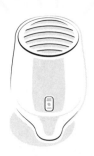

Like nebulizing diffusers (page 32), fan diffusers rely on air movement, rather than heat, to diffuse essential oils; unlike nebulizers, which use vibration, fan diffusers consist of a motor-driven fan that blows air over or through a pad holding the essential oils. Because fan diffusers use a pad to hold the oils, the viscosity of the oil makes no difference — unlike nebulizing diffusers, which are easily clogged by viscous oils. This makes fan diffusers perfect for thicker oils, like vetiver or myrrh, that cannot be used in a nebulizing diffuser.

One downside of a fan diffuser is that the force of the air can be so great that the oils are diffused too quickly. The speed of diffusion depends mostly on the volatility of the oils being used, of course: the lighter the oil, the faster it will dissipate. Delicate florals, for example, are wasted in a fan diffuser. It is best to use this type of diffuser only for heavier oils.

Did You Know?

There are tiny fan diffusers available for personal spaces, and larger models capable of scenting up to 1,000 square feet (93 m²) of space.

Plug-In Diffusers

Plug-in diffusers use electricity to create heat, which diffuses the essential oils. It is best to use this type of diffuser for no more than 10 to 15 minutes at a time; longer than that, and the heat may start to corrupt the oils.

Home Plug-Ins

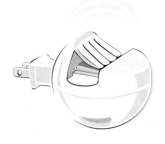

These little devices have become rather ubiquitous over the last several decades, mostly due to big chemical companies like SC Johnson, the maker of Glade products. The trouble is that the brand-name versions with prefilled cartridges use synthetic scents. Far from being therapeutic, synthetic scents have been implicated in a number of health conditions, including many hormonal imbalances, as they are known endocrine disruptors. (See page 7 for more information about synthetic scents.)

Thankfully, there is another type of plug-in diffuser that uses a pad instead of a prefilled cartridge to hold the essential oils, and this type allows you to use essential oils in place of synthetic scents. The pad rests on a small warming strip that is activated only when the device is plugged in. The heat, while mild, is still warm enough to change the chemical profile of the oils, especially if the device is left plugged in for too long, so be sure to set a timer when using one.

I like plug-in diffusers for their ease of use — the pad is held in place by widely spaced bars, and you don't have to remove the pad to add oils. When you want to change scent profiles, replacement pads are available and are easy to change out.

I use a plug-in diffuser in my clinic between patients, for 5 minutes or so, just to freshen the room. Because I often diffuse oils therapeutically during treatment (always with a nebulizing diffuser, described on page 32), I avoid using strong scents in the plug-in, as they could interfere with the subsequent treatment.

Clear the Air
A drop of cooling peppermint oil in the summer or bright grapefruit oil in the winter is a nice way to clear the air.

Car Plug-Ins

Car plug-ins work exactly the same way as home plug-ins, but are designed to fit into a car's lighter socket. I recommend them quite frequently for people who suffer from anxiety or tension while driving, and they can really help reduce the tendency toward road rage (although no essential oil will address the underlying issues that can lead to it).

During pollen season, try using an oil or blend that helps reduce allergy symptoms, so you can get from one place to another without having a sneezing fit or any other distracting allergic reaction.

As with the home plug-ins, do not run these devices for too long, or the heat may corrupt the oils.

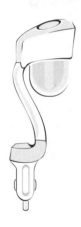

Electronic Diffusers

Electronic diffusers are more expensive than the other options, but deliver a more therapeutic diffusion. Most aromatherapists, including me, consider them to be the best diffusers, by far. If you're using essential oils for therapeutic effects, definitely consider investing in one of the models described here. They are well built and last a long time — several years at least.

Nebulizing Diffusers

Hands-down the best option for therapeutic applications, nebulizing diffusers use compressed air or ultrasonic waves to break down essential oils into aerosolized micro droplets. These micro droplets stay suspended in the air much longer than larger droplets, as the weight of each droplet is so low. As you might expect, when oils stick around longer, they work longer. Nebulizers are thus both more effective and more efficient than other types of diffusers. They are best used with a timer, as they are so effective it is really easy to overdo it — 10 to 15 minutes of use is usually sufficient.

Nebulizing diffusers that are attached to a pump (like one you might use in a fish tank) use compressed air to create a stream of air from the tip of the device. Those that use ultrasonic waves create a fine mist, but unlike the ultrasonic diffusers described below, these devices do not use water; the mist is pure essential oils.

The one major drawback to nebulizing diffusers is that they cannot handle viscous oils, which tend to clog them up. If you are using a blend of many oils that includes just one drop of a viscous oil, it may be okay, but in general, it is best to avoid thicker oils altogether or risk ruining the diffuser — an expensive mistake!

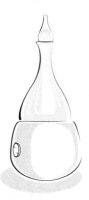

Bacteria Battlers

Nebulizers quickly disperse enough essential oil into a room to effectively reduce airborne bacteria by up to 70%. As such, they are the diffusers of choice for use in clinics and treatment rooms. Using one in a sick room at home has the advantage of treating both the sufferers and those supporting them through the sickness.

Ultrasonic Diffusers

Ultrasonic diffusers (also called cool mist diffusers or cool mist humidifiers) use ultrasonic waves to break water and essential oils into tiny particles, creating a fragrant mist that hovers in the air, mostly around the diffuser. They can be used anywhere you might use a humidifier.

In addition to *looking* really cool, the mist *is* cool, as no heat is used. An ultrasonic diffuser is perfect for helping to fragrantly cool an area (for example, an outdoor seating area in summertime), although their effect on temperature is slight. They also add moisture to the air, so they are more appropriate in places with very low natural humidity levels. If you live in a region prone to mold or mildew, adding more moisture to your environment might not be such a good idea.

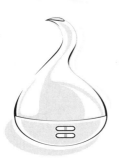

A Word of Caution

Some ultrasonic diffusers cannot be used with citrus oils, as these can damage certain types of plastic. If using citrus oils is important to you, be sure to buy an ultrasonic diffuser that specifically says it can handle them.

Personal Diffusers

Unlike diffusers designed to fill a room with scent, personal diffusers can be used discreetly, without affecting the environment of those around you. Many personal diffusers are small — easily worn or slipped into a pocket to be used as needed. Some are passive, meaning they diffuse scent without any action on your part, while others may need a lid removed or a quick pump to activate the scent.

Scent Jewelry

There is a wide variety of scent necklaces and bracelets available, in many different decorative styles. What they all have in common is a built-in well for a felt pad or other absorbent material to rest in. You simply add a drop or two of your desired essential oil or blend to the pad and tuck it into place in the necklace or bracelet. They are very easy to adapt to whatever blend circumstances call for, as you can easily change pads for a different scent anytime you like. A quick swipe of rubbing alcohol over the jewelry between scent profiles will ensure that the scents remain pure, with no cross-contamination.

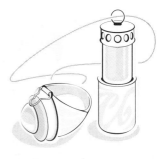

If you prefer your scent to be a bit more contained, there is another necklace style that consists of a tiny bottle with a stopper that can be removed as needed. These are often beautifully crafted pieces with beaded bands that attach the bottle to the necklace chain. (If you are crafty, you can easily make one at home with some copper or silver wire wrapping.) Be careful with this type of necklace, though — every time you remove the stopper, there's a chance of drips or spills, and some essential oils can stain clothing.

Be on the lookout for "poison" rings. These rings have a tiny compartment that opens, and were purportedly once used to carry around small amounts of poison to spike an enemy's drink or food. These days, instead of wearing such a ring to make someone else ill, we can use the little chamber to store a tiny piece of cotton or felt, and add a drop of essential oil!

Antique Lockets

I have seen scent necklaces made with antique lockets, where, instead of pictures, a little pad sits in the frame. If you love antiques, keep your eyes peeled for these old lockets, often available at very affordable prices.

Scent Vials

Scent vials are perhaps the easiest way to carry and sniff a scent. Simply make the blend you would like to use right in the bottle, and carry it with you. A dram bottle is a good size — these tiny bottles usually hold about 20 drops of an essential oil or blend. The lid often has a little black applicator stick attached, which is helpful if you need to add a drop of scent to a cotton ball, for example.

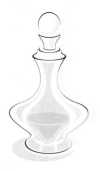

Although these bottles are glass, they are so small they are quite difficult to break! However, to be on the safe side, consider carrying the vial in a little cloth bag or purse. I often carry several vials in one bag. If you decide to do this, be sure to differentiate the blends from each other. I add a dot of nail polish to the bottom of each vial, but a colored thread wrapped several times around each bottle and tied off tightly will also work. (Now you just have to remember what the colors stand for!)

Pet Collar Diffusers

There are pet collars on the market with little passive diffusers built right in. My personal take on these is that they are fairly unethical, and can be downright dangerous. Dogs and cats have an incredible sense of smell that they rely on to navigate their world. Essential oils can be disorienting to animals, and some can cause liver damage, as many animals do not have the enzymes needed to metabolize essential oil molecules. (Keep in mind that these molecules are readily absorbed into the bloodstream through the skin.)

In an article in the June/July 2011 edition of *Animal Wellness* magazine, author Vicki Rae Thorne offers reasonable suggestions for the safe use of essential oils with pets. If you decide to use one of these collars on your pet, be sure to read her suggestions first. This is one category where I suggest purchasing a commercially available collar, as safeguards are (or should be!) in place to protect your pet.

For information on safely diffusing essential oils in a home with pets, see page 77.

Spritzers

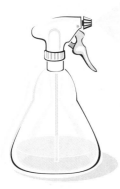

These are super-easy to use and so affordable! Glass spray bottles are best, as the inert material will not interact with the essential oils. Simply fill the spritzer bottle about two-thirds full with filtered or distilled water, then add several drops of your blend or single oil. Spritzes are best used up within a week or less, so make small amounts.

Before spritzing, shake the bottle well. Most essential oils will float on the surface of the water, and shaking will temporarily emulsify them into the water. If you do not shake right before spritzing, each spritz will contain less essential oil — except for the last few spritzes, which will be quite intense!

Don't spray more than a few pumps at a time, at most, and avoid spraying directly into your eyes — or onto your skin, for that matter, if you are using potentially irritating oils like clove or peppermint. You'll also want to avoid certain surfaces, such as plastic or wood, because the spray may leave a residue or damage the surface. It is best to spray up into the air, then allow the mist to slowly settle. You can also spray cotton balls, tissues or other disposable items when you want the scent to be more localized.

Smelling Salts

Salt is a wonderfully receptive material. When essential oils are added to salt, they are absorbed into the salt's structure, which slows their release. It is important to use the right kind of salt, however. Fine table salt will not work well, as the oils will tend to make it clump. Kosher salt or coarse sea salt is best. Himalayan salt crystals also work well.

A Word of Caution

This section does not refer to medical smelling salts, which are not actually salt (sodium chloride), but a chemical compound that releases ammonia, causing a physiological reaction — a sharp inhalation that brings oxygen to the brain. Medical smelling salts are designed to wake up an unconscious person and should not be confused with essential oil smelling salts.

Smelling salts are quite easy to make at home: all you need is a container to put them in. It is better to avoid plastic, as some essential oils (citrus and evergreens in particular) will cause plastic to deteriorate rather quickly. A small glass or metal salve jar is the perfect size and shape.

In theory, the more salt you add to the container, the longer it will diffuse. Just add several drops of your chosen single oil or blend to the salt in the container, place the lid on the container and gently shake.

Whenever you feel the need for a quick blast of your chosen scent, simply open the lid and sniff. Don't feel you have to stick your nose in the jar! In fact, it is much better to sniff from a few inches away, after the scent has opened up a bit. Replace the lid as soon as possible to prolong the effectiveness of the smelling salts.

The limitation of smelling salts is that the scent profile is set — they cannot be reused with other blends unless the original oils are part of the new blend. I like to throw used salts into a bath when I am finished with them (see page 24). The heat of the water releases the scent even when it is no longer perceptible in the container.

Experiment with Lecithin

Some people like to add a touch of lecithin, a natural emulsifier, to a spritzer, but I find it does not work as well as I would like and often leaves clumps in the bottom of the bottle. Feel free to experiment!

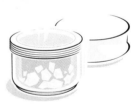

Did You Know?

Do not be tempted to add essential oils to a Himalayan salt lamp! The warmth of the lamp will diffuse the oils rapidly, like a candle-heated diffuser (see page 23), and the oils will break down the salt crystals over time.

Inhalation Sticks

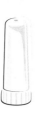

These devices (also called inhaler sticks or aroma sticks) are represented in the retail market by products like Olbas Inhaler and Vicks Inhaler. They consist of a plastic tube that holds a dense cotton roll called a wick stick. Essential oils are added to the wick, and strategically placed vent holes allow the scent to be inhaled directly from the tube. The tube is screwed onto a base, and a plastic cover keeps the scent from dissipating too quickly.

Inhalation sticks are very popular at the moment, and it is easy to find the components to make your own (see Resources, page 207). I have found that they work best for addressing imbalances of the respiratory system (sinus congestion, for example), as they direct the oil exactly where it is needed.

If there is any drawback to these devices, I would say it is the fact that most are made of plastic and are considered "disposable," as the oils will inevitably break down the plastic. There are aluminum and glass versions, which are preferable, but they are usually more expensive. On the other hand, the glass has the advantage of being easy to clean so that no trace of the previous scent can be detected, which means that they can be reused again and again with different scents. In the long run, a reusable device may well end up being less expensive than a disposable one!

Personal Nebulizing Diffusers

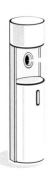

It is now easy to find battery-powered personal nebulizing diffusers about the size of a pack of cards or even smaller. These handy devices, which contain a small reservoir for water and oils, start to diffuse as soon as they are opened and do the job in half the time of other personal diffusing devices, such as inhalation sticks.

A personal nebulizing diffuser is fantastic for addressing respiratory imbalances if used properly. The best approach is to inhale the blend from a short distance, especially when you're first using the device.

They do have a few drawbacks: the batteries make them a bit heavy, the battery life seems to be fairly short, and the reservoir needs to be filled often to avoid running the diffuser on empty.

The quality of these little diffusers can vary greatly, so be sure to research the options before buying one.

Did You Know?

It is very important to thoroughly clean your personal nebulizer on a regular basis. Make sure it is completely dry before storing it.

A Word of Caution

A nebulizing inhaler is a similar device used for respiratory disorders, like asthma or COPD, as it allows the medication to get deep into the lungs. Do not use your nebulizing inhaler to diffuse essential oils!

Vaporizing Pens

Inspired by e-cigarettes, these relatively new devices are specifically designed to allow oral inhalation of an essential oil or blend. The essential oils are diluted in a base oil (usually coconut oil), and the device gently warms the blend to diffuse it into the lungs.

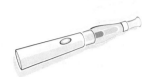

There is nothing inherently wrong with inhaling essential oils directly into the lungs; in fact, many people use other types of diffusers to do exactly that — especially nebulizing diffusers, which are used in respiratory therapy. But because these devices are so new, the jury is still out on whether they are a good idea.

Smoking Cessation

Because vaporizing pens mimic a cigarette in shape and function, they may not be the best choice for ex-smokers and people trying to quit smoking, as they encourage the hand-to-mouth association that you're trying to break. For smoking cessation, you might be better off using another type of diffuser with an oil blend that both benefits the lungs and helps reduce the urge to smoke.

Topical Treatments

When you start to read the section of the book on improving your health with essential oil diffusion (pages 80–180), you will notice a recurring theme of boxes with information on topical treatments. You might wonder why a book on diffusing essential oils mentions topical treatments at all. It is important to understand that a large percentage of the scent molecules volatilize out of essential oils, which is why we are able to detect when someone is wearing a scent blend. The boxes describe how to turn an essential oil blend into a topical treatment to enhance the diffusion experience. For example, if you are suffering from a sore throat and a cough, diffusing the appropriate blend will help with the cough, while applying the same blend (always diluted in a base oil!) to the throat will help soothe the pain.

Skin treatments are another area in which diffusion and topical treatments can be paired for maximum benefit. Steam diffusion is a fabulous way to reduce blemishes, for example, and the same oil blend can be used as a spot application.

Wherever I suggest a topical treatment, I provide directions for combining the essential oil blend with a safe and appropriate carrier substance, such as a fixed oil, aloe or vinegar, to ensure that the blend is safe for topical use.

Essential Oil Basics

It has taken me many years of study and experimentation to understand the "natures" of essential oils, and I will share some of what I have learned in this chapter. But if your actual experience with the oils differs from how I have suggested they might work, then your response overrides all theoretical information. Your personal response is the last word in terms of what oils to use and how to blend them. If an oil does not address your imbalance in the way this book suggests it might, try other oils or blends instead.

Choose Organic

Only fresh, high-quality oils made from organically grown or ethically wild-crafted plants processed in an organically certified lab or distillery should ever be used in aromatherapy — that is, if you are addressing an imbalance. If the purpose of diffusing is to scent your space, it is sometimes okay to use oils that do not adhere to these stringent guidelines, although it is still preferable.

An important point to remember: if you do not actively enjoy the scent of an essential oil or blend, it will be less effective. A disliked scent can actually be counterproductive, as emotional responses to scent deeply influence us on many levels. Remember the last time you smelled something distasteful to you, and recall your reaction. Not healing! If you do not like a blend, start over! The blends in this book use very small amounts of essential oil specifically so you can experiment and not lose too many drops of these precious healers.

As with any other potent healing agent, essential oils can be misused and can be harmful if used incorrectly. Be sure to read "Diffusing Essential Oils Safely" (page 76) before embarking on your journey with these wonderful agents of change.

The most important suggestion I can make, though, is to have fun — and share the love with others whenever possible!

How Aromatherapy Works

To a large degree, aromatherapy works by affecting mood or inducing a different sensation. The shift occurs in the neuroendocrine system, which is constantly receiving and sending chemical signals that change our state of being by shifting levels of hormones and other chemicals. Communication within the body is utterly dependent upon this system, and nearly all of our physiological functions rely on chemical signaling. Hormones play an enormous role here, along with other factors like minerals and amino acids.

So how do essential oil molecules make their way into the neuroendocrine system? The molecules released by the oils are extremely small and light, and are quite active when released. These molecules are easily drawn into the nose by the slight draft our breathing creates. Once inside the body, they travel through various structures, each perfectly designed to accommodate the molecules on their journey. The molecules land on receptor sites on nerve endings, triggering a release of information to the olfactory bulb.

Here is the really interesting part: the olfactory bulb is part of the brain. This means that physical information from outside the body has entered the body and directly touched the brain. This is a very unique situation — the brain does not, for the most part, like to be touched. But it happily, and instantly, responds to scent molecules, conveying messages primarily to the glands (the pituitary, the hypothalamus) and to the brain stem. Because the resulting chemical cascades are closely allied with the brain stem, the oldest part of the brain, many of the reactions we have to scent are reflexive and do not require higher thought.

Did You Know?

Hormones are the body chemicals most impacted by essential oil molecules. The smell of bergamot, for example, has been shown to stimulate the brain to generate the neurotransmitters serotonin and dopamine.

How Essential Oils Are Created

Essential oils are created from different parts of a plant — rose petals are used for rose essential oil, for example, and fennel seeds for fennel essential oil. Some plants offer up different oils from each of their various plant parts. For example, sweet orange essential oil is made from the rind of the fruit, neroli essential oil is derived from orange blossoms, and the green twigs and leaves of the bitter orange produce petitgrain essential oil.

Essential oils are extracted from the plant by the following methods:

Did You Know?

The essence of the plant is captured through various means, but primarily through a process known as distillation.

Steam Distillation

Distillation appears to have arisen in many parts of the world at around the same time. The Greek alchemists in Alexandria worked extensively with the process of evaporation and condensation, and passed the tools of this process on to the Arab world, where the technique was preserved.

To this day, steam distillation is the most common means of extracting essential oils from plants. Here is how the process works: the plant material is loaded into the top section

Did You Know?

The creation of the distillation device commonly called a "still" is usually attributed to the Medieval scholar Ibn Sina (known in the west as Avicenna) in the 10th century; however, Maria Prophetissa wrote about using an alchemical still in the 1st century, long before Ibn Sina spoke about distillation.

of a distillation device. The bottom is filled with water that is then heated to produce steam. As the pressure builds, the steam is forced through the plant matter, which liberates the essential oils. The mixture of water and oil is then passed through a coil immersed in cold water, which forces the two to separate. From the coil, the separated liquid passes into a receiving vat. The final step is removing the lighter essential oils floating on the surface of the water. The water that remains is also used in aromatherapy. It goes by several names, but is most commonly called hydrosol.

Expression

Expression is the technique used for plants that store their essential oils in the skin of the fruits they produce. These are mostly the citrus oils, such as lemon and grapefruit. It is quite easy to access these essential oils — if you have ever peeled an orange and seen the fine mist spraying from the peel (which seems, inevitably, to end up in someone's eye), you have expressed an essential oil. For mass production, a large press is used.

Enfleurage

Enfleurage is an old technique that has been mostly abandoned, except by the most dedicated natural perfumers, as it is a long and labor-intensive process designed to remove scent molecules from delicate flower petals that cannot withstand steam distillation. During this process, a layer of solid fat is painted onto a smooth, flat surface, such as marble or glass. Flower petals are meticulously laid down on the fat and left for a day or two. When all the scent has been removed, the spent flowers are stripped off and a new layer is added. This procedure may be repeated dozens of times before the fat is washed with alcohol to separate the essential oils. After the alcohol is allowed to evaporate, the remaining substance is called an absolute.

Sourcing Essential Oils

Always look for the purest essential oils processed from organic plant matter when using them for therapeutic aromatherapy. This is the only way to ensure that you are promoting good health with these medicinal substances.

Chemical Extraction

Nowadays, most absolutes are created by chemical extraction. Hexane is commonly used as a solvent and, despite being quite volatile, never completely leaves the absolute. It is nearly impossible to find organically certified absolutes, but because the substances left behind in this process are mostly used in perfumery and not for therapeutic aromatherapy, it is not an issue for our purposes.

In recent years, a newer method, carbon dioxide (CO_2) extraction, has offered exciting possibilities. When gaseous CO_2 is put under enough pressure, it becomes a liquid that is particularly good at liberating essential oils. An added bonus is that many compounds poorly extracted by water (steam distillation) — substances like waxy fatty acids, for example — are easily accessed by CO_2 extraction. This adds depth and richness to the resulting oils. The best part, however, is that when the process is finished, the pressure is released and the CO_2 returns to its gas form, leaving behind a pure essential oil with no residues.

Choosing Essential Oils

There are many different systems for understanding how essential oils should be chosen, from traditional usages to a detailed breakdown of their chemical constituents. If you are interested in learning about these subjects, I have recommended some excellent reference books in the Resources (page 206).

I wanted to share a more intuitive way to determine which oils to use and how to blend them. This system is based on recognizing where an essential oil comes from, as the part of the plant used to distill the oil often gives you a clue about how best to use it:

If the essential oil comes from:	Examples:	It may help with:
Bark	Cinnamon	Protection at the surface
Flowers	Inula, rose	Euphoric, connecting
Fruit	Black pepper, lemon	Revitalizing, uplifting
Leaves	Basil, peppermint	Refreshing, cleansing
Resin	Frankincense, myrrh	Overall protection
Root	Ginger, vetiver	Grounding
Seeds	Anise, fennel	Calming, storing resources
Wood	Cedarwood, sandalwood	Centering, deepening

As you learn more about essential oils and begin to use them, you will start to appreciate on a more instinctive level the connections between an oil's source and its effect. But keep in mind that your personal response to an oil is always the most important determining factor in how to use it. If you respond to a particular floral aroma by becoming more grounded, then for you, that oil is grounding.

When it comes to blending oils using these ideas, get creative! It may seem contradictory to feel scattered and overly grounded at the same time, but consider something like bipolar disorder, where brain fog and depression are often experienced simultaneously. Another example is the flu, which leaves us feeling vulnerable at the surface and depleted of energy on a deeper level. Cinnamon and fennel oils would address both issues, and a drop of lemon oil would help us feel more alert.

Commercial oil blends tend to address only one issue: uplifting or sedating, for example. But the human experience is often more complicated. Understanding the oils allows you to blend them for more complex situations. For more information on blending, see page 75.

Ammi

(Ammi visnaga)

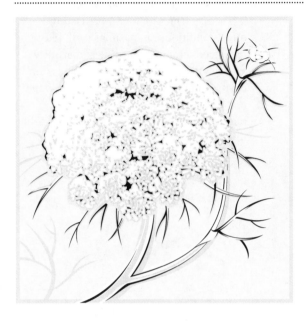

Also called khella, this oil is so strongly bitter and sharp, it is best used very sparingly. It does have a nice earthy, woody tone to it as well, which helps moderate the bitterness of the first note. Ammi is mainly used for asthma or other constrictions, but its scent is so strong, it absolutely must be tested first, as it could trigger a reaction. Many who use this plant choose the capsule form rather than the oil. However, I have found the oil to be incredibly effective at reducing spasm and constriction anywhere in the body. In addition to treating bronchial spasm, it is also used for both spasm and sclerosis of the blood vessels, for example. Ammi essential oil is warm and moisturizing, and tends to move energy down in the body.

Angelica

(Angelica archangelica)

Reminiscent of anise or fennel, this plant has long been used as a digestive aid. Its scent is peppery and herbaceous, with a slightly spicy note. The essential oil is warming and drying, and because of this can be very helpful with cold, damp digestive issues, such as diarrhea. Angelica oil tends to bring increased circulation of vitality.

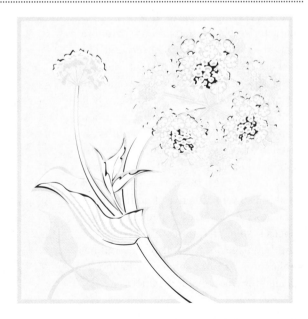

Anise

(*Pimpinella anisum*)

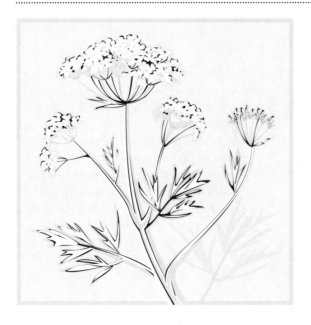

As with angelica (page 43) and fennel (page 53), two oils that share a scent profile with anise, the benefits of this oil are mostly upon digestion. Specifically, it is antispasmodic. It can be used in other conditions of spasm as well, like menstrual cramps, but it has an affinity for the gut. The main notes are sweet and clean, and the sweet scent is immediately recognizable. Anise oil is neutral in temperature, meaning it may be applicable to either hot or cold symptoms.

Basil

(*Ocimum basilicum*)

Because basil is so ubiquitous in cooking, its scent has been known to immediately induce a craving for pesto! It is characterized by an herbaceous high note, supported by a bit of spicy bitterness. The final note is sweet and persistent. Basil oil is slightly warm but tends to move heat in the body, rather than add to it. It can help draw heat from the head to the lower body if applied to the feet, for example. It is an excellent choice for issues of the nervous system, whether they manifest emotionally or as an issue with the nerves themselves. Basil is also very effective at addressing circulatory imbalances, especially of the venous system, like varicose veins. Holy basil (see page 56) is a subspecies and has similar actions, although it may be more specific for emotional imbalances.

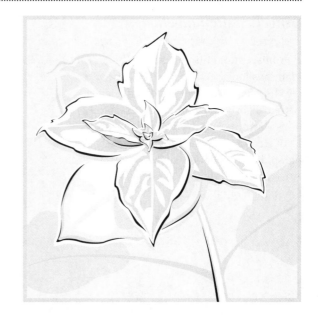

Bay Laurel

(Laurus nobilis)

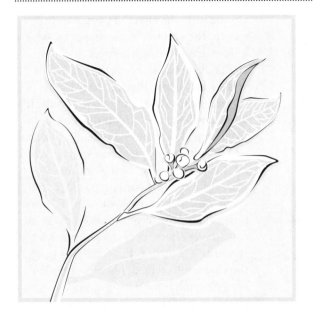

Very fresh, green and spicy, with a touch of camphor at the end, bay laurel is specific for stagnant lymph, helping to encourage circulation of the lymphatic fluid, but is helpful for all stagnation, including respiratory fullness or stuck phlegm. It is understood to work by cooling heat and encouraging the moistening of thickened fluids.

Bergamot

(Citrus bergamia)

Bright, fresh, citrusy and sharp, bergamot is the scenting agent used to make Earl Grey tea, so its scent is quite familiar to many people. The oil is used in blends for everything from respiratory to digestive imbalances. It is also helpful in skin conditions, especially where oiliness and dryness coexist. This oil should never be applied to the skin before you go out in the sun, as it is phototoxic, leading to greater damage from ultraviolet rays.

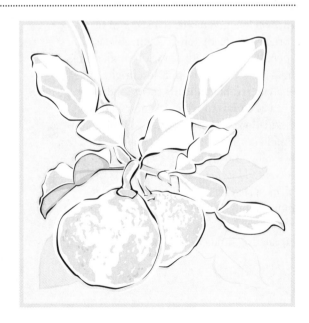

Black Pepper

(Piper nigrum)

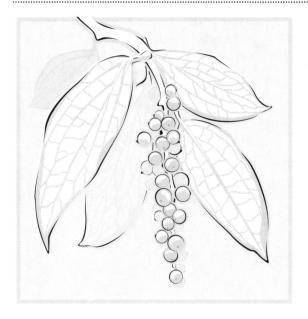

Considering the effect of pepper in the mouth, the scent of black pepper oil is milder than one might expect. It can be characterized as spicy and bright, sharp and slightly bitter. Black pepper is my favorite oil to add to circulation blends. It is an excellent rubefacient, reducing pain, increasing blood flow and generally perking up the system. As might be expected, the oil is hot and can be drying, making it perfect for treating persistent cold, damp conditions, like postnasal drip. At the same time, adding it to blends for sinus congestion can be very effective, as the sharp scent can stimulate the flow of thin secretions to open the sinuses. As a food, black pepper can act as a catalyst for the anti-inflammatory effects of ginger or turmeric, for example, and I have found the essential oil to be anti-inflammatory as well.

Black Spruce

(Picea mariana)

Like all evergreen oils, the scent of black spruce is immediately recognizable as such. Black spruce has a fruity undertone, but is primarily balsamic and bright. It is an incredibly uplifting scent, and is used in blends to increase energy and circulation. It is often added to topical liniments. The oil can be somewhat warming, mostly as a side effect of increased circulation. The addition of black spruce to a blend can increase its moisturizing properties — again, mainly because it helps increase the flow of all circulating fluids in the body.

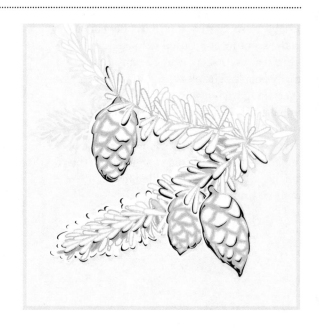

Blue Chamomile

(Tanacetum annuum)

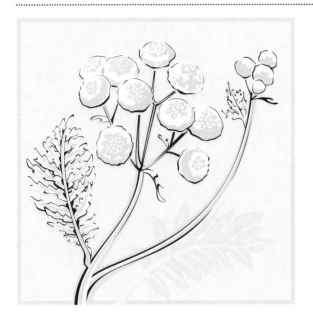

Also known as blue tansy, this bright blue oil is sweet and fruity, fresh and rich. It is also very dense — a little goes a very long way. It is cooling to hot conditions and inflammations of all kinds. Consider blue chamomile wherever there is heat, itching or irritation, not just for allergies, bites and stings, but for any irritation of the skin. If you want to add a touch of fruitiness to any scent, try blue chamomile in tiny amounts.

Cacao

(Theobroma cacao)

Cacao essential oil is less chocolaty than you might imagine, but the scent is definitely characteristic. Warm, balsamic, bitter and slightly earthy, cacao adds depth and richness to any oil blend. In this book, I've used it to help with coffee or sugar addiction. It blends well with Peru balsam, rose, sweet orange, cinnamon and, of course, vanilla!

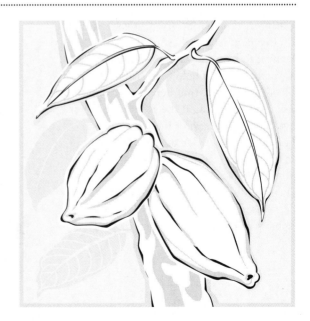

Cardamom

(Elettaria cardamomum)

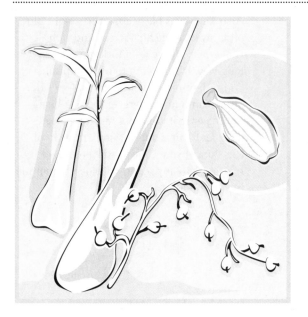

Cardamom oil is warm, spicy, balsamic and fruity, and some people have suggested it contains eucalyptus notes. Cardamom seeds are used for digestive imbalances in many traditions, and that's how I have used the essential oil in this book. It is a very nice addition to any blend that needs depth and brightness at the same time, and is an interesting addition to aphrodisiac blends as well.

Carrot Seed

(Daucus carota)

Carrot seed oil has a very strong scent that is often characterized as "peculiar," but I find it to be woody and rootlike. It is such a wonderful oil to help with issues of the blood and toxicity that I encourage you to use it even if you find the scent odd. It has a particular affinity for the liver and can help clear toxins. Carrot seed oil is neutral in temperature and quite moisturizing, an effect achieved through its ability to move stagnant fluids. The general direction of action is up, as it helps bring fluids to the upper part of the body quite effectively.

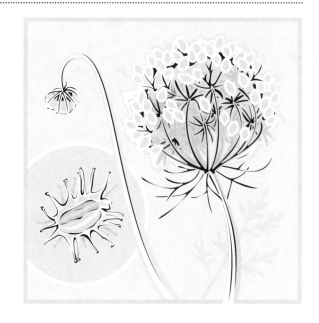

Cedarwood

(Cedrus spp.*)*

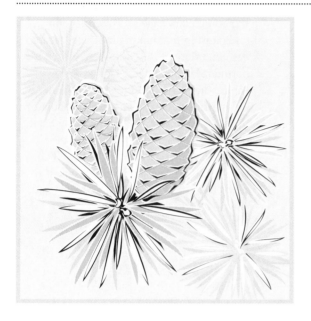

Camphoraceous and sweet, but also woody, cedarwood oil's scent is grounding and calming, and can help support you through trials, both emotional and physical. Cedar of Lebanon was used for the doors of churches for many years, and for this reason, the smell is still somewhat ecstatic for some. Cedarwood essential oil is warming and slightly drying, and moves energy up to the chest and head.

Cinnamon

(Cinnamomum verum)

The very recognizable scent of cinnamon essential oil is described as warm, dry, spicy and sweet. In terms of therapeutic action, the oil is actually quite hot and dry, and tends to draw energy down and in, making it quite tonifying in general. Because of its strong association with cooking, especially sweets, some people find that it satisfies food cravings.

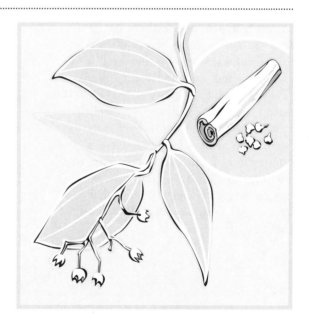

Clary Sage

(Salvia sclarea)

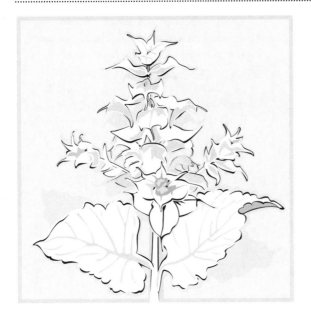

In action, clary sage oil is both cooling and moistening, making it perfect for hot, dry conditions. It has a marked effect on hormonal imbalances, like hot flashes. Interestingly, the oil tends to draw energy up, but this action seems to self-regulate by also encouraging energy to move back down. Because of this, I describe clary sage as having a circulating action. The scent is both sweet and herbaceous; it tends to hang around (it's tenacious) and can be a little bittersweet.

Clove

(Syzygium aromaticum)

Primarily used as an anesthetizing agent in aromatherapy, a tiny bit of clove oil can also add an exotic note to any blend. It is a hot oil and can burn tissues if used undiluted. It is drying, as well, and moves energy from the outside in, so it can help when there is cold in the interior of the body. The scent has been described as fruity, although I personally do not get that hit. It is fresh, somewhat sweet and very spicy. Like carrot seed, it is an oil that has been called "peculiar," which I interpret to mean exotic.

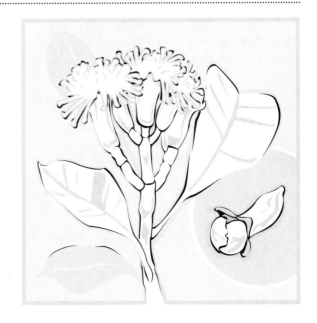

Cypress

(Cupressus spp.)*

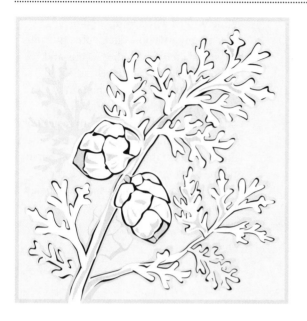

Like a breath of fresh air, the fruity sweetness of cypress oil can revive a dull mind better than any other oil. The oil is cooling and moistening — in my experience, it achieves this by helping to circulate and redistribute stagnant fluids — and can therefore be very helpful in urinary imbalances. In addition to fruity and sweet, the scent is somewhat balsamic, and can be delicate. I find it to be quite tenacious, especially if used alone.

Eucalyptus Citriodora

(Eucalyptus citriodora)

Like all the eucalyptus oils, eucalyptus citriodora is warming and drying, perfect for damp, cold conditions like postnasal drip. This species, as the name implies, carries citrus notes and is specifically beneficial for cold in the joints, such as osteoarthritis. It is also strongly antiviral. Eucalyptus citriodora essential oil tends to move energy up and out, helping to circulate warmth where it is needed. In addition to being citrus-like, the scent is fresh and somewhat rosy, with a slightly balsamic finish.

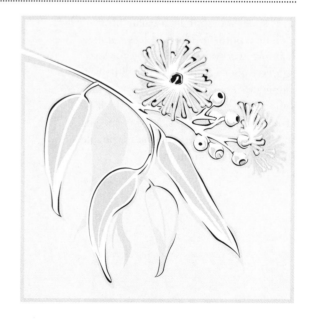

Eucalyptus Globulus
(Eucalyptus globulus)

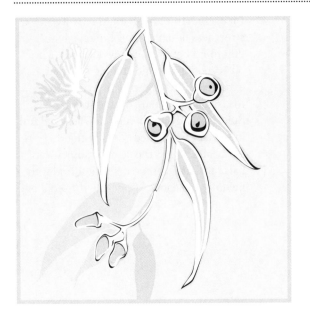

While it's just as warming and drying as other eucalyptus oils, eucalyptus globulus has a much more camphoraceous and medicinal odor than the others. I find it to be the most universally helpful of the bunch as well, effectively addressing a wide range of imbalances, from respiratory to muscular. Like all the eucalyptus oils, it is strongly antiviral. It is somewhat harsh and may be inappropriate for the very young (consider eucalyptus radiata, below) or the elderly (try eucalyptus citriodora, page 51).

Eucalyptus Radiata
(Eucalyptus radiata)

This species is similar to eucalyptus globulus, but is milder and less harsh. It is also warming and drying, but less aggressively so, and its scent, while still camphoraceous and medicinal, is a bit softer. Like all the eucalyptus oils, it is strongly antiviral. Consider this species for children over one year and for people in a weakened condition.

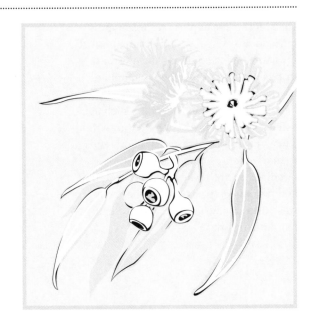

Fennel

(Foeniculum vulgare)

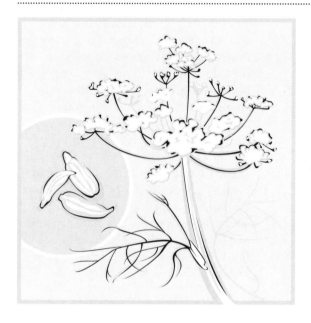

Commonly used in foods to aid digestion, fennel is very sweet, somewhat earthy and a bit peppery or spicy. Most people find that its first note, the sweetness, overrides all the others. It is characterized by a licorice-like scent, which means it is not as useful for people who do not like that flavor. (It has been shown again and again that an oil is less therapeutically useful if the user dislikes the scent.) Fennel essential oil is warming and fairly neutral in its moisturizing effects. Like all oils that help with digestion, it moves energy into the center.

Fir

(Abies spp.*)*

A high-quality fir essential oil will almost always have a rich, fruity note reminiscent of jam. In fact, the term "jammy" is often used to describe fir oil! Once you get your first whiff of a good fir oil, you will immediately relate to the jam note. Therapeutically, the oil is cooling and moistening, and helps to redistribute fluids in the body, typically by moving energy up rather than down and out. It can be very useful with edema of the lower body. The scent, in addition to being jammy, is sweet and quite balsamic, like many of the evergreen needle oils.

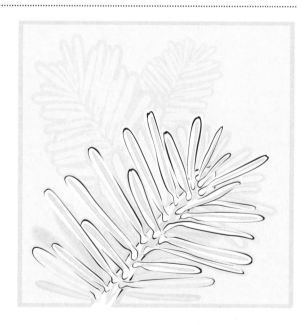

Frankincense
(Boswellia spp.*)*

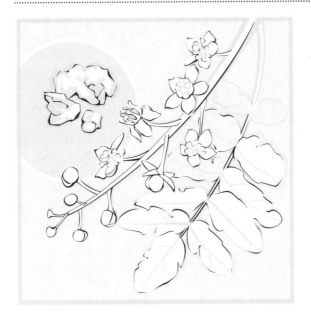

Just the word "frankincense" can evoke a sense of ecstasy in people from many different cultures around the globe, as this oil (or the resin from which we get it) has been used in religious rites and spiritual practices for a very long time. It is an excellent oil to consider when training the mind to break habits or learn a large volume of information quickly but well. It is also used in many skin-care blends, as it helps to generate healthy tissue. The scent has been described as similar to unripe apples, but to my nose it is more peppery and balsamic, with a rich, sweet-woody finish. Frankincense is my favorite oil by far.

German Chamomile
(Matricaria chamomilla)

I rarely use this oil, as blue chamomile (page 47) can be used for many of the same imbalances and is much less expensive. However, a small amount of German chamomile is in some cases more beneficial than a much larger amount of blue chamomile. German chamomile is slightly more specific for digestive complaints, while blue chamomile may be faster-acting against heat and inflammation. German chamomile is intensely sweet and herbaceous, with the same fresh, fruity, apple-like undertones as its more affordable cousin. It is also just as intense — a tiny amount goes a very long way.

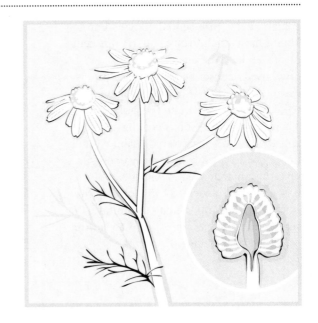

Ginger

(Zingiber officinale)

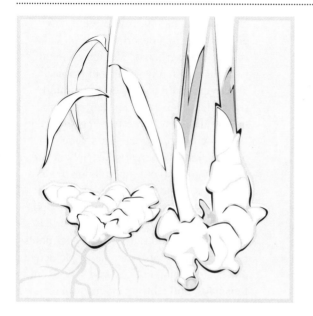

As might be expected, ginger essential oil is hot and dry. Rather than leaving the body feeling desiccated, however, ginger will help get things moving by circulating stuck energy. Its scent is also characterized as woody, spicy and fresh, with some citrus notes. The scent is tenacious, finishing out with a balsamic floral note long after it has lost the fiery spice of the first note.

Grapefruit

(Citrus x paradisi)

Grapefruit may be one of the most delicious essential oils I know. It is incredibly fresh and uplifting without being overwhelming. The oil is considered to be neutral in temperature, making it useful for many situations, although some people find it a bit cooling. It can be somewhat drying and tends to move energy down. Like the source material (grapefruit rind), the oil's scent is fresh and intensely citrusy, with a sweet undertone. Some people detect bitter notes as well.

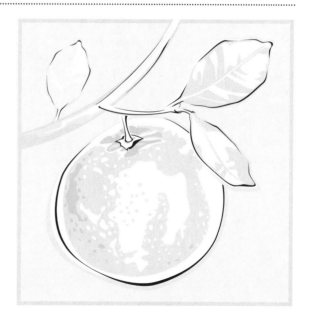

Helichrysum

(Helichrysum italicum)

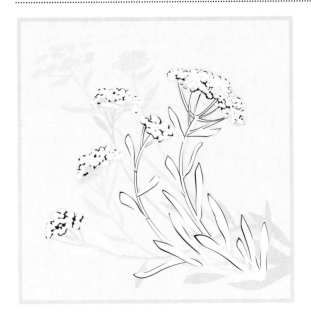

This oil may be my "if you could have only one oil on a desert island" pick. It is such a powerhouse! Helichrysum oil is healing on many levels, but primarily acts to circulate energy evenly around the body. It is neither hot nor cold, and neither drying nor moisturizing, and can therefore be appropriate for a wide variety of imbalances. Energetically, helichrysum oil moves in and out, up and down (all directions, basically!), and is excellent for clearing stagnation of all types — blood, lymph, qi or energy. The scent profile is sweetly fruity and rich, with deeper notes reminiscent of honey. Some people detect a delicate tealike note as well. The scent is tenacious, and a little helichrysum oil goes a long way.

Holy Basil

(Ocimum tenuiflorum)

Like its more plebeian cousin, holy basil (also known as tulsi) is herbaceous, sweet and persistent, but this variety also carries a slightly more aniseed note. While it can be used in all the same ways you might use regular basil (page 44), I find holy basil to be more appropriate for mental and emotional imbalances, and for settling the spirit.

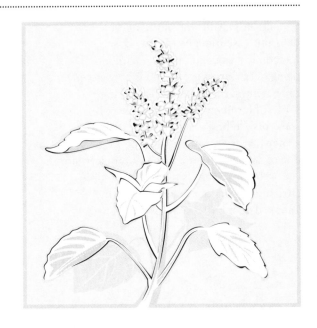

Hyssop Decumbens

(Hyssopus officinalis var. decumbens)

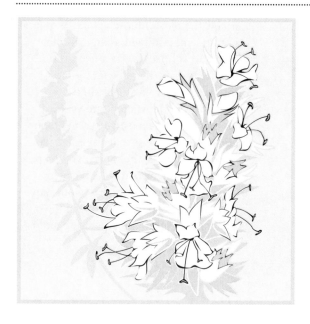

This oil is not terribly common, and is perhaps a bit limited in its uses, but when it is needed, there is no other oil that works in quite the same way. It helps to open bronchial tubes very effectively, without being aggressive. It is important to note that no other variety of hyssop is either safe or effective, so be sure to buy only essential oil made from this subspecies. The effects of hyssop decumbens oil are somewhat cooling and drying. It helps move energy down and out, which makes sense, as many respiratory problems are related to shallow breathing (or what, in Chinese medicine, we call reverse qi: when qi is going the opposite direction from the way it naturally flows). Hyssop decumbens oil is very sweet and somewhat camphoraceous, with an overall warm note that soothes irritated nerves and tissues.

Inula

(Inula graveolens)

Inula is probably underutilized and is less well understood than many essential oils. This incredible oil is usually a brilliant emerald green, the result of reactions between the oil and copper in the still. It is a fantastic mucolytic, meaning it breaks down mucus. In addition, it reduces bronchospasms. Together, these two properties make inula incredibly effective against most respiratory imbalances. The oil is fairly neutral, so it can be used for both cold and hot conditions. The fragrance is very bright and sharp, and also somewhat herbaceous. Use with caution; inula may be sensitizing.

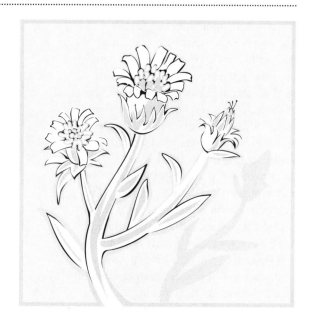

Jasmine

(Jasminum spp.*)*

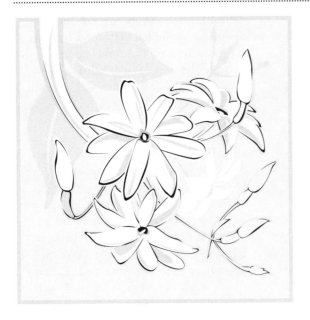

Perhaps the most intensely floral, euphoric scent known, jasmine has an extremely long history of use. It was a necessary ingredient in any floral blend for most of human history — at least in those parts of the world where it grows. In aromatherapy, it is mostly used in libido blends, to enhance sexual arousal. Like all euphoric florals, the movement is up to the head and beyond, which is why using too much jasmine for too long can lead to feeling dopey or high. Jasmine oil is generally neutral in temperature and is somewhat moisturizing.

Juniper Berry

(Juniperus spp.*)*

Most people immediately associate the deeply rich and warming scent of juniper berries with a high-quality gin, as these berries are a main ingredient in that spirit. Juniper berry essential oil is warming, but unlike many warming oils, it is also moisturizing. It achieves its moisturizing effect primarily by redistributing fluids, making it very useful in edema — especially of the upper body, as the energetic movement of this oil is primarily downward. The scent is fresh and slightly bitter, but also very aromatic. Like black spruce or fir, it is one of the woody-sweet scents we tend to associate with winter. I like to use juniper berry oil in a sick room, as the volatile molecules are incredibly effective at combating airborne microbes.

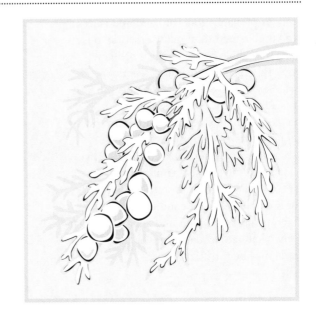

Lavender

(*Lavandula* spp.)

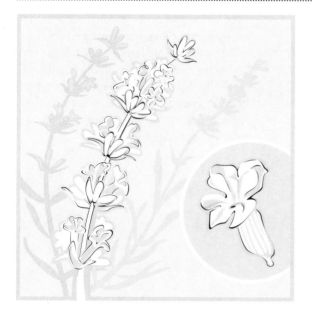

Without question, lavender oil is the best known, the most familiar and, in my opinion, the most overused of the essential oils. It is also one of the most widely effective oils against a whole host of imbalances, which accounts for its popularity. The oil is fairly neutral to somewhat cooling. It can help to moisturize tissues and supports systemic circulation of energy. The scent is sweet, floral, herbaceous and slightly balsamic, with a woody undertone that tends to linger.

Lemon

(*Citrus* x *limon*)

Instantly familiar in most parts of the world, the scent of lemon is at once sunny and bright, fresh and somewhat sweet, slightly sharp and a little bitter. Lemon essential oil is both cooling and drying, thanks to its astringent properties (that pucker when we eat lemon is a good clue). Lemon oil is an excellent disinfectant — in conjunction with ultraviolet rays from the sun, lemon can successfully eradicate most microbes from surfaces; as a result, it is often found in cleaners.

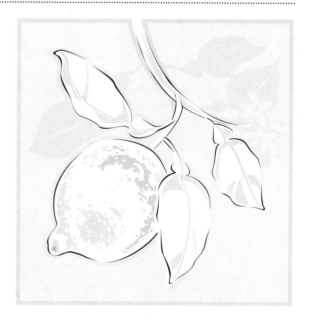

Lemongrass

(Cymbopogon spp.)

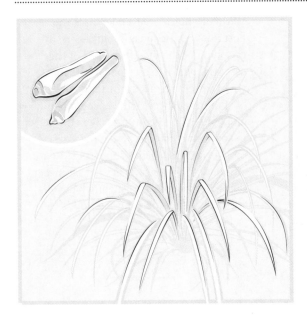

Like lemon (page 59), lemongrass is both cooling and drying, but lemongrass acts more by dispersing fluids (rather than astringing tissues, as lemon does). This oil generally moves energy inward and may help dry boggy tissues at the surface. The scent is both strongly lemonlike and grassy, with an appealing fresh note.

Marjoram

(Origanum majorana)

Slightly sweeter and more camphoraceous but very similar in scent to its close cousin oregano (page 63), marjoram essential oil is also cooler and less harsh than oregano oil. It is somewhat drying and helps descend energy, making it useful for addressing imbalances such as high blood pressure or vomiting. In addition to the notes listed above, marjoram is warm, spicy and a little bit woody.

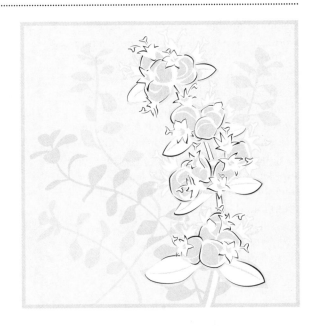

May Chang

(Litsea cubeba)

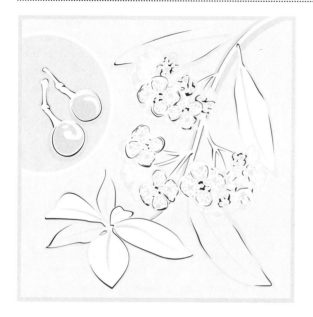

Distilled from the tiny berries of a type of laurel, may chang is very lemony and sweet, fresh and fruity. It is bright, like lemon, but softer and sweeter on the whole. It is less drying than the other citrus-like oils, and more fugitive, meaning the scent does not linger like the more tenacious aroma of lemon or orange. It makes an excellent substitute for any citrus when you are blending florals, as it will not overwhelm the more delicate flower notes. May chang tends to circulate energy rather than draw it in or down, as many of the citrus and citrus-like essential oils do.

Melissa

(Melissa officinalis)

While most of the citrus and citrus-like essential oils are helpful for calming and centering, melissa — also known as lemon balm — takes the cake. It has been used in whole herb form for hundreds of years to help students focus in school, and is extremely helpful with vacillating moods and bipolar disorder. The oil is generally cooling and drying, and helps to circulate energy, one of the reasons it is so helpful with seesawing emotional states. The scent is fresh, light, citrus-like and slightly floral.

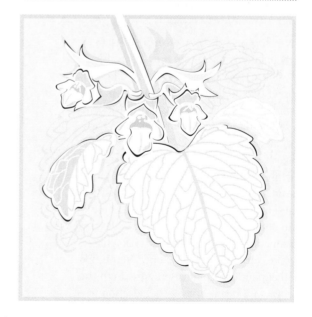

Only a very small amount of melissa is needed in blends, which is fortunate because this essential oil is incredibly expensive. If you are lucky enough to have a compounding pharmacy near you, it may be possible to obtain melissa oil in a dilution. Many studies have shown that this oil is actually most effective in a very dilute state: 1:99.

Myrrh

(Commiphora myrrha)

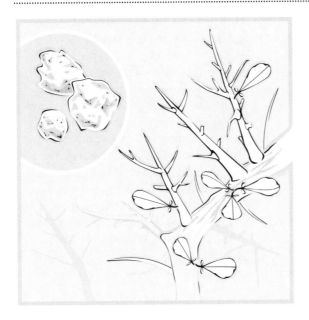

An evocative scent that is familiar to many people thanks to its heavy use in religious and spiritual rituals, myrrh is the other half (with frankincense) of the most famous blend known. Like frankincense, myrrh is neutral in temperature and can be used for both hot and cold imbalances. It is somewhat moistening and quite antimicrobial — the oil is often used in mouthwashes to eradicate bacteria and help heal gums. As with many of the oils used in rituals, myrrh can facilitate up-down communication, both within the body and in the environment, meaning it can help us be more aware of our surroundings. The scent is warmly balsamic, quite sweet and somewhat spicy.

Neroli

(Citrus aurantium)

Neroli is one of three essential oils generated by *Citrus aurantium*, in this case from the orange blossoms. The other two are bitter orange oil, from the rind of the fruit, and petitgrain (the least commonly used of the three), from the small twigs. Neroli is one of the most exotic and evocative scents I know — one whiff and I am instantly transported to Andalusia or Morocco. The scent is sweet, and heady without being heavy. There is an odd note in this oil that some describe as metallic but that, to me, feels a bit more mineral, like wet stone. Neroli, like all euphoric oils, moves energy up to the chest and head. It is a good addition to blends designed to encourage heart-mind connection.

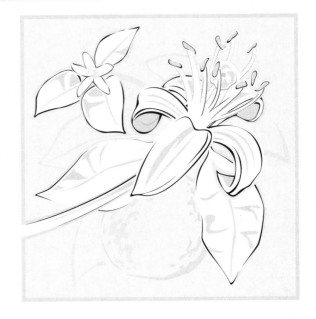

Oakmoss

(Evernia prunastri)

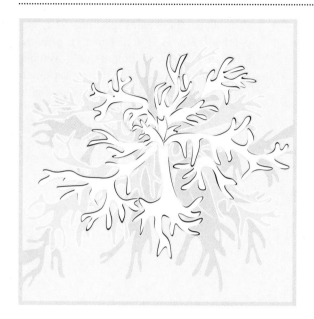

Distilled from lichen, oakmoss may be the oddest oil I know in terms of its scent profile: it literally smells like a forest floor! Rich and earthy, dense and very much like humus, oakmoss finds its way into many blends for men, as it grounds more spicy scents, being extremely tenacious. I was once asked by a young friend to make a blend that smelled like her grandfather's woodshop, and oakmoss was the first ingredient I selected. It is both antiseptic and anti-inflammatory, making it useful in wound blends.

Oregano

(Origanum vulgare)

Strongly medicinal, oregano essential oil is dramatically antimicrobial, beating out some conventional pharmaceuticals in its ability to eradicate certain strains of bacteria. The scent is camphoraceous, woody, warm and "dry" — a note that is immediately recognizable once encountered. Oregano oil is neutral to cooling, and quite drying. The energetic movement is more descending and can help draw energy out of the head.

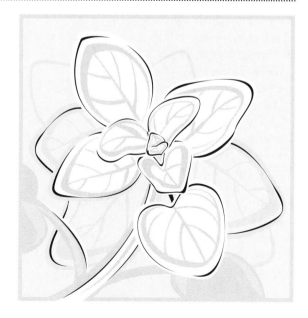

Patchouli

(Pogostemon cablin)

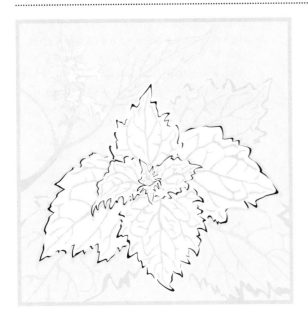

Poor old patchouli. Cheap, young (or raw) patchouli was used so heavily in the 1960s, it became known as "hippie smell." Which is a shame, as aged patchouli is an extremely rich and aromatic oil, sweet and spicy with beautiful balsamic notes. It has been used for a very long time in skin-care blends, as it is amazingly effective at balancing dry, tired skin. As might be expected, patchouli oil is warm and moisturizing, and draws energy inward to assist with repair.

Peppermint

(Mentha piperita)

An immediately recognizable scent, peppermint oil may well be the most universally accepted essential oil. If you want to use an oil in a public place, consider peppermint — I have never had a single negative response to it in all my years of diffusing. Peppermint is an interesting oil, as it is both cold and hot, making it very effective at circulating energy, especially at the surface; peppermint oil in skin-care blends moves energy like nothing else I know. It is also somewhat drying, making it helpful at reducing boggy inflammation. The scent is fresh, strong, grassy-minty, sweet and very clean.

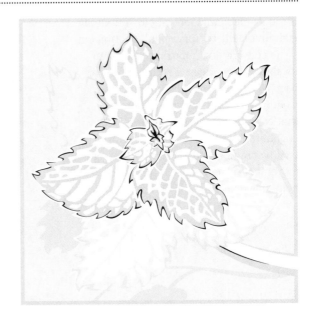

Peru Balsam

(Myroxylon pereirae)

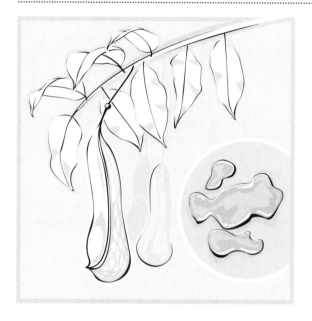

Sweet, rich and tending toward cocoa-like, the scent of Peru balsam can be quite heady, and a bit overwhelming for some. Use the oil in small amounts. Dense, viscous oils like Peru balsam tend to be very beneficial to the skin. It is neutral to warm, but does not seem to exacerbate conditions of heat. As an excellent demulcent, Peru balsam can provide topical protection for any tissue irritation, such as hemorrhoids or ulcers.

Pine

(Pinus spp.*)*

Pine is a scent that is typically associated with cleanliness, thanks to generations of pine-based cleaners. The oil is somewhat antiseptic on surfaces, especially against airborne microbes. Pine essential oil is neutral both in temperature and in its moisture-regulating function, making it extremely useful for a wide variety of imbalances, and particularly respiratory conditions. It tends to circulate energy back to the body, so it may be helpful for imbalances that leave you feeling exhausted. The scent is slightly sweet but mostly woody, with a balsamic undertone vaguely reminiscent of turpentine.

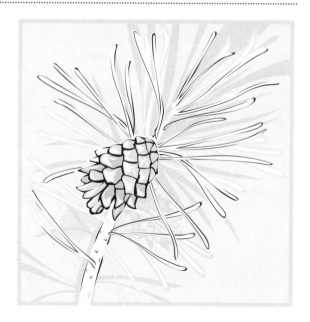

Ravintsara

(Cinnamomum camphora)

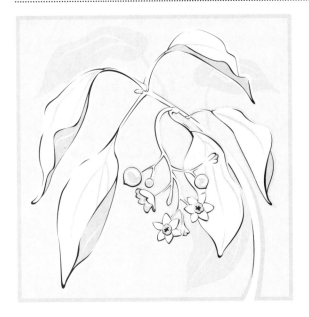

Like eucalyptus (pages 51–52), ravintsara is most helpful with viral infections. It seems to be especially useful with the mucous membranes of the mouth and throat, and can both prevent and reduce throat infections if used at the first sign of a tickle. Like juniper berry (page 58), it is a good oil to consider using in the sick room to reduce airborne microbes. Ravintsara is neutral in both temperature and moisture regulation (despite coming from the same family as cinnamon, which is very hot), and can assist with up-down movement of energy, making it a good choice for issues involving stagnation. The scent is strong and penetrating, with a woody nature.

Red Mandarin

(Citrus nobilis)

Red mandarin is the citrus oil to consider first when you're treating energy imbalances in children. Small amounts will focus and calm frenetic energy, and slightly higher amounts can be quite sedative. The scent is citrusy and very sweet, with a somewhat floral note at the end. As with many of the citrus oils, red mandarin helps move energy in, which is in part why it is so effective at calming and centering.

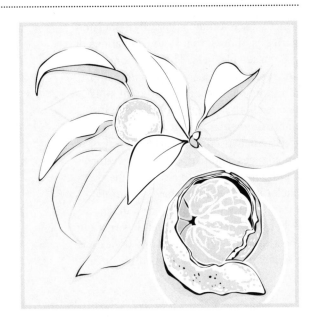

Roman Chamomile

(Chamaemelum nobile)

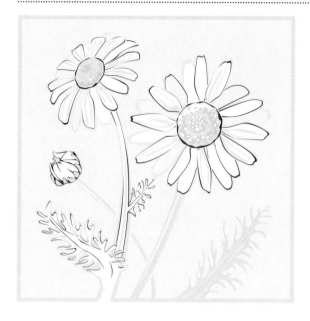

Unlike its German cousin (page 54), Roman chamomile does not turn blue when steam-distilled, so the color is one of the easiest ways to ensure that you are using an oil from the correct species. Although somewhat anti-inflammatory, Roman chamomile really shines as an antispasmodic agent, with an affinity for the chest and gastrointestinal tract. However, consider this oil for any blend to treat spasms, as it will work in many different systems. The scent is sweet, like German and blue chamomile (page 47), but more herbaceous and less fruity, and the tealike notes are much more pronounced in Roman chamomile. The scent is also less tenacious than the other chamomiles. In terms of energetics, this oil is warming and moistening, and generally moves energy up and out.

Rose

(Rosa spp.)

Like patchouli, rose is a scent that has been typecast: many people associate it with little old ladies. But that's not a fair association unless those little old ladies are vibrant and sensual, seductive and exotic — which, to be honest, is often the case these days! Rose oil's scent profile is nearly impossible to describe, as there are so many varieties of roses being distilled these days, but in general they all tend to be rich, warm and sweet, with some spicy notes. In addition, rose is, of course, the epitome of the floral note. The oil is often used in libido blends for its cooling, moisturizing properties. These properties also make it very useful in skin-care blends. Many people find rose oil to be centering, calming and uplifting, and some describe it as spiritually grounding.

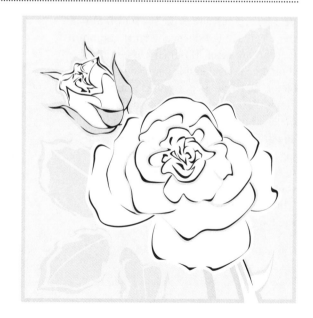

Rose Geranium

(Pelargonium graveolens)

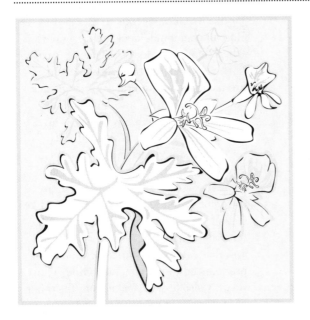

Rose geranium (also simply known as geranium) is much more earthy than its noble sister the rose (page 67). In addition to its lightly rosy nature, there are herbaceous and rootlike, earthy notes in rose geranium essential oil, occasional citrus hits and sometimes a peppery note. These days, the oil is primarily used in blends to balance women's cycles and in skin-care blends. It is also strongly antifungal. Rose geranium oil is neutral both in temperature and in its moisturizing effects, meaning it can be effective for both oily and dry skin. The energetic movement tends to be downward and inward — in other words, tonifying and reparative.

Rosemary

(Rosmarinus officinalis)

Very few scents will wake up your brain the way rosemary does: one sniff and brain fog starts to clear. Rosemary essential oil should be considered for any cognitive blend. Its fresh, woody notes, reminiscent of a walk through an evergreen forest, make it one of my favorite essential oils. It is warming and drying, perfect for cold, damp conditions. As it tends to move energy up, it is a good pick for something like lower limb edema, in which cold and damp have settled into the lower extremities.

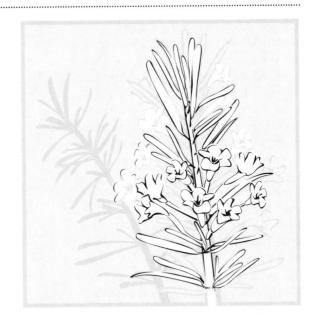

Sage
(*Salvia officinalis*)

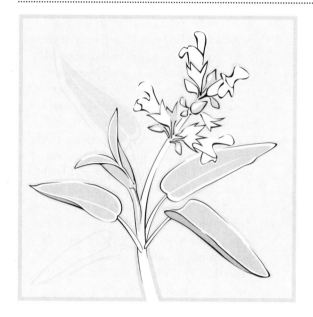

Sage essential oil from *Salvia officinalis* is far less commonly used than its distant cousin clary sage (*Salvia sclarea*), and is used for very different sorts of imbalances. While clary sage (page 50) is gentle, and is essential for women's health imbalances, sage is much more aggressive and must be used with a judicious hand; I cannot remember ever using more than one drop of sage in any blend. Having said that, sage oil is incredibly effective at what it does, which is primarily to dry up secretions. It is found in natural antiperspirants and may help to dry up breast milk after weaning. It is also useful, in tiny amounts, to help break down scar tissue. Sage oil is neutral to warm in temperature, and draws energy into the center. The scent can be described as strongly herbaceous with a spicy note, and somewhat camphoraceous.

Sandalwood
(*Santalum album*)

Sandalwood oil is cooling and especially good at moving stagnant fluids. It is used for urinary imbalances and in skin-care blends and natural perfumes. The scent consists primarily of spice and wood notes, with a soft, slightly musky middle and a bittersweet finish.

It is important to stress that Indian sandalwood should not be used unless it is proven to come from an ethically harvested source. The sandalwood industry has very nearly driven this amazing tree to extinction, a terribly sad reality we as consumers need to remedy. There are now sandalwood plantations in other parts of the world, like Australia, that grow and harvest very sustainably.

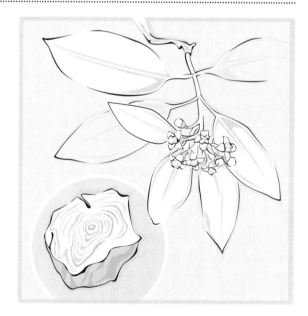

Spikenard

(Nardostachys jatamansi)

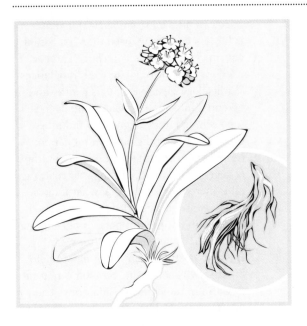

One of the oils mentioned in the Bible, spikenard (also known as nard) is a scent both rare and peculiar. Best described as heady, the oil is also, oddly enough, quite heavy. There are sweet and woody notes, but the primary overriding feel is animalic, which basically means musky. I am not partial to actual musk sourced from animals (and the harvesting practices can be terribly cruel), so spikenard, which I love, is a very helpful oil to have on hand for that particular note. Spikenard is warming and moisturizing. It moves energy down, making it indispensable for grounding and very useful in sleep disorders. It is one of the few oils I think of as actively sedating.

Sweet Orange

(Citrus sinensis)

Sweet orange essential oil is pressed from fresh orange rind and is immediately identifiable as such. If you have ever peeled an orange, you have inadvertently released essential oils — the fine spray that squirts into the air is pure sweet orange essential oil. Like many of the citrus oils, it is cooling and drying. Sweet orange oil tends to move energy up to encourage a reciprocal downward flow, which is part of why it can be either uplifting or sedating, depending upon the amount used and the length of your exposure to it. Most people, if breathing in a lot of sweet orange oil for a long time, will start to feel sleepy, even if they at first found it stimulating. The scent is bright, fresh, sweet and, of course, citrusy.

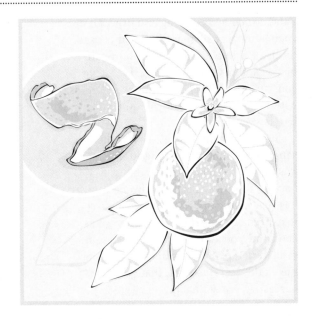

Tangerine
(*Citrus reticulata*)

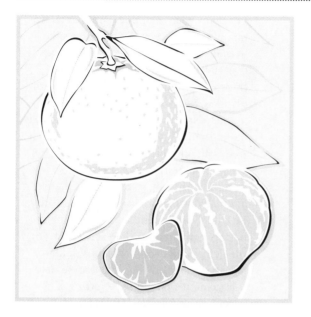

Tangerine is a bright citrus option that is slightly sharper and more sour than sweet orange (page 70), with a slightly bitter note at the end. The oil is cooling and moving, and like many citruses, is either uplifting or calming, depending upon dosage.

Tarragon
(*Artemisia dracunculus*)

Primarily used for digestive complaints, tarragon essential oil is extremely effective against spasms of the gastrointestinal tract, including spasms of the esophagus (commonly called hiccups). It is strongly antimicrobial and has anesthetic properties as well, making it especially useful in treating the pain of spasm. The oil is warm and slightly drying. In terms of energetic action, it tends to draw energy in to the center of the body (like most essential oils that are effective for gut problems). Interestingly, tarragon oil also helps to increase circulation, perhaps by moving the blood at the core rather than at the surface.

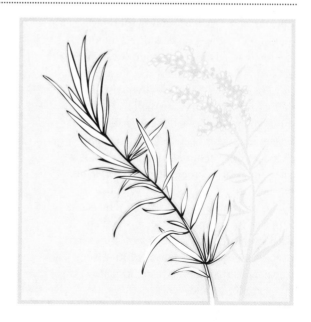

Tea Tree
(Melaleuca alternifolia)

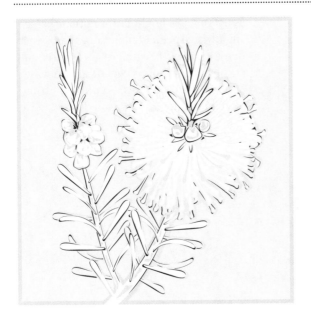

For many years, tea tree essential oil was ubiquitous — it was nearly impossible to find a commercial blend that did *not* contain this useful oil! Unfortunately, this high demand led to a flood of hastily distilled, inferior tea tree oil in the market. Now that the trend is fading, it is easier to find high-quality oils again. Tea tree is an oil that should probably be on everyone's shelf, as it is useful for so many things. (Although, to be honest, there are many oils I could say that about!) It is strongly antimicrobial and healing, a perfect combination. The scent is strongly medicinal and camphoraceous, but also somewhat spicy, with a turpentine note that some people find off-putting. The oil is cooling and drying, and tends to move energy up to the chest.

Thyme
(Thymus vulgaris)

Like oregano (page 63) and marjoram (page 60), thyme (also called red thyme) is strongly medicinal in action. It can be harsh and irritating, so it is best used in tiny amounts. I like to use thyme in a footbath to give it time to mellow before it hits the nose. It is a hot and drying essential oil, and needs a judicious hand or it can overwhelm. Having said that, it is incredibly antimicrobial and, like oregano, has been shown to be highly effective against certain bacterial strains. The scent is powerful, warmly herbaceous and spicy, with sweet undertones. It is best to reserve thyme essential oil as a heavy hitter for imbalances that are not responding to applications of milder oils.

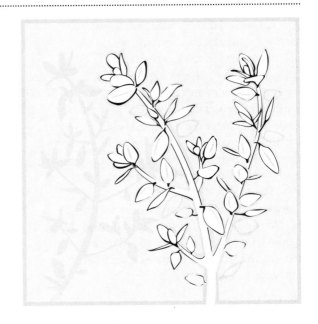

Thyme Linalool

(*Thymus vulgaris* ct. linalool)

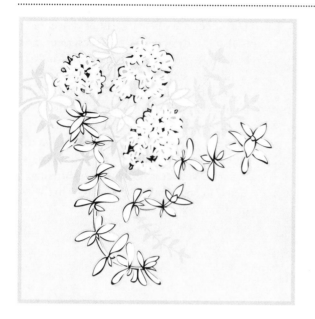

Unlike its stronger cousin, thyme linalool is mild in both action and scent. It is gentle enough to be included in skin-care treatments, something I would never do with regular thyme (page 72). The warm, slightly spicy and herbaceous notes characteristic of all thyme essential oils are softened by rich, sweet citrus notes. Thyme linalool oil is more neutral in temperature, and is surprisingly moisturizing where red thyme is drying. It tends to move energy down, which can help with heat in the face, for example.

Vanilla

(*Vanilla planifolia*)

Instantly recognizable and evocative, vanilla's scent is sweet, warm, rich, exotic — and yummy! The oil is used in this book primarily to soften and sweeten blends, especially in the section on addiction (page 81). Vanilla essential oil is warming and consolidating, meaning it can help with feelings of fragmentation or scattered thoughts, and is very grounding.

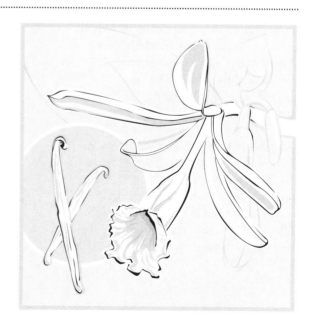

Vetiver
(Chrysopogon zizanioides)

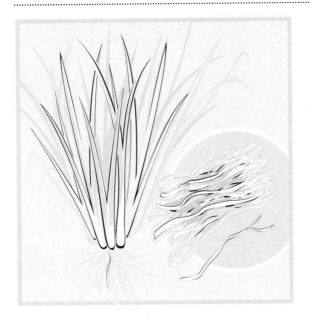

The sweet, very heavy scent of vetiver oil is also woody and earthy — described by many as rootlike. It is definitely an acquired taste! Made from the roots of a grass that typically grows high on the Pampas of South America, the oil is useful for connecting head to feet; that is, when you are feeling ungrounded and spacy, this oil can help bring you down to earth. Vetiver is cool and moisturizing. Use it in any blend that threatens to fly up and away!

Ylang Ylang
(Cananga odorata)

This is one of the sweetest florals I know; in fact, ylang ylang can be sickly sweet if used in too high a concentration. It may be slightly balsamic and is highly diffusive, readily dominating small spaces and taking a long time to fade. I never use more than one drop in any blend. Ylang ylang essential oil is commonly found in libido-enhancing blends or anywhere one is looking to add a euphoric note. It is primarily cooling and moisturizing, and is occasionally used to treat irritated skin. Like all of the euphoric floral essential oils, it primarily moves energy up.

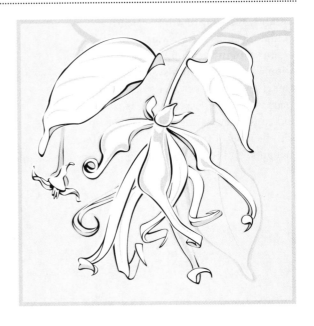

Using Single Oils vs. Making Blends

I often use single oils. Sometimes, a single is exactly what a particular situation calls for. If the effects of a single oil cover all the actions you are looking for, consider using it as a stand-alone scent.

On the other hand, oil blends can definitely address a wider range of imbalances. In some cases, blends include oils that help "drive" the formula to a particular part of the body, by taking advantage of the affinity an oil can have for a system or region of the body. For example, florals go up to the head and beyond. If you are feeling low and stagnant, floral blends can help get you out of the slump. In contrast, feeling ungrounded calls for essential oils whose primary action is to descend. Some oils that have an affinity for both the urinary and the respiratory systems can be directed to one or the other of these systems by the supporting oils added to the blend.

Practically speaking, using single oils is simple. Open a bottle and give it a sniff! Then pay attention to your response. If you find the response useful, try diffusing a drop of that oil. Passive diffusion (see page 20) is a good place to start. Monitor your response as it changes — does the oil start out energizing but end up being sedative (as can happen with sweet orange oil, for example)? Do you love it at first sniff but find it cloying after some time has passed (as is my experience with some of the more heady florals, like ylang ylang)?

When blending essential oils, I do it right in the bottle. The heavy-walled blue, green or brown glass bottles in various sizes work really well and are designed to accept a restrictor cap (an insert that fits the top of the bottle and reduces the size of the opening, allowing you to closely monitor the amount dispensed). These bottles and caps are now widely available from many different distributors. I usually use 5 mL bottles, as I rarely make more than that at one time —

Try Dilution

If you find a single oil to be overwhelmingly heavy or strong, consider diluting it with a base oil or blending it with essential oils that cut through that heavy scent.

About the Blend Ratios

The number of drops indicated in the blend formulas in Part 2 are *ratios*, not necessarily concrete amounts. For example, if you are preparing the Wake Up! blend from the "Fatigue and Low Energy" section (page 95), you *could* just prepare a bottle with 3 drops of bergamot oil, 1 drop of black spruce oil and 1 drop of helichrysum oil, or you could make a larger batch of the blend using the ratio 3:1:1. In other words, for every 3 drops of bergamot oil, you would add 1 drop of black spruce and 1 drop of helichrysum.

Making
Topical Blends

Making
Topical Blends

When making a blend for topical use, I like to add the essential oils to the bottle first, then top them up with the suggested amount of base oil (see page 198) or other base material. A small funnel is useful, but watch carefully, as it is easy to overfill the bottle if you are not paying close attention. If you add the essential oils last, be sure to stir carefully with a disposable bamboo skewer or toothpick so they are well incorporated into the base material.

Ingestion

Avoid ingesting essential oils except under the supervision of a trained aromatherapist. Since the advent of essential oil products designed to be ingested, the number of adverse reactions has risen precipitously.

it's potentially wasteful, as my needs may change before the blend is used up. However, if you find yourself creating a lot of blends in base oils (see sidebar), you may prefer the 15 mL bottles.

It is not always necessary to mix a blend in a bottle. If you are trying out a blend in a humidifier, for example, you can add the recommended number of drops of the blend directly to the well. Keep in mind that the longer the oils are exposed to the air, the more they will volatilize; be sure to start the treatment as quickly as possible after exposing the oils.

Keep it simple. Complicated blending with more than a few oils is not necessary. As you will notice, I have used just three oils for every blend in this book. Three is a great number to choose, as it allows for more specific variations on a theme. For example, skin rashes can be hot, dry or oozing. The first two oils in a blend can be generally beneficial for rashes, while the last one addresses the heat, dryness or ooze.

Diffusing Essential Oils Safely

It is important to keep in mind that essential oils are very potent healing agents and must be treated with respect. There is a great deal of misinformation about essential oils, but a few guidelines can help you use them wisely.

First, it is rarely necessary to use more than a few drops of an oil or blend. Really. One drop is often all that is needed to effect change. This may be difficult to believe, but overusing oils in either volume or frequency is both wasteful and potentially dangerous. Start with the smallest possible amount and build up *if needed.*

Many people are extremely sensitive to inhaled scents, whether from natural or synthetic sources. If you have known sensitivities or a respiratory condition, proceed with caution when using an essential oil for the first time. It may be best to have someone quickly open and close the bottle some distance away from you and wait a minute to see if the scent molecules cause you any distress.

Use extreme caution when diffusing essential oils in any of the following situations:

- **During pregnancy:** It is best to get the advice of an aromatherapist if you or anyone in your home is pregnant. Many essential oils are contraindicated during pregnancy.

- **Around children:** If you have children in your household under the age of two, consult an aromatherapist before diffusing essential oils. Make sure children cannot gain access to your essential oil bottles; keep them safely stored in a place where your kids can't find them.

- **If you have a seizure disorder:** Anyone with a history of a seizure disorder should be extremely careful when using essential oils, as they have been reported to trigger seizures.

- **If you are allergic to salicylates:** Some essential oils, such as wintergreen and birch, contain salicylates. I have not included any of these oils in this book.

Although this book is mainly about diffusion, essential oils can also be applied topically, and many of the blends in this book suggest topical treatments that can be used in addition to (or instead of) diffusion. If you decide to use essential oils or blends in this way, please keep the following precautions in mind:

- **Patch test:** Be sure to do a patch test first. Apply one drop of the blend, diluted in a base oil, to an area of thicker skin, like your shoulder or knee. If there is any reaction, discontinue use.

- **Photosensitizing oils:** Be aware that certain essential oils, when applied to the skin, will cause photosensitization, meaning that if the sun's rays fall on that area of skin, they will cause cellular damage. The

Clean Up Spills

Remember to immediately wipe up any spills when using essential oils and blends. Many oils are caustic and will deteriorate a lot of different materials, especially anything plastic. Porous surfaces will readily absorb essential oils, and it may be difficult to eradicate the scent from those surfaces. If an old spill has a lingering odor, a paste of baking soda and hydrogen peroxide may remove it. But be aware that this combination has a bleaching effect — use with caution!

Pets and Essential Oils

Using essential oils on and around pets is tricky. Certain blends are useful to help keep ticks and fleas away, or to help heal hot spots, for example. On the other hand, dogs and cats have an exquisitely acute sense of smell that they rely on to navigate their world. Overwhelming their sense of smell with essential oils seems like a bad idea. Further, there have been many reported cases of neurological damage to pets, especially cats, from being doused in essential oils.

Never douse anything in essential oils.

Having said that, extremely small amounts of oils or blends are probably okay, especially for larger pets. If using a blend to deter pest infestations, add the essential oils to your pet's collar instead of the skin. If treating an area of skin, be sure the oil is well diluted in a base substance. If your pet starts acting strangely after being exposed to essential oils, remove the oils immediately — take off the collar and/or bathe your pet if necessary.

As with children, make sure pets cannot access your essential oil bottles.

most common photosensitizing oil is bergamot, but all of the citrus oils may result in damage. Become informed about which oils are safe in the sun!

- **Mucous membranes:** Avoid allowing undiluted essential oils to make contact with any mucous membranes, such as the vagina, anus or the lining of the nose or mouth. It hurts! Some essential oils, especially those containing aldehydes, can damage sensitive tissues.

Storing Essential Oils

Because of the reactivity of many essential oils, it is important to store all oils in a cool, dark place, at least. Certain oils are best stored in the refrigerator — especially oils high in aldehydes, like oregano, cinnamon or lemongrass — because cold slows oxidative damage. Aldehydes are very electron-active oils and will readily bond with the oxygen introduced each time a bottle is opened. Oxidation not only renders an oil basically useless for therapeutic purposes, but also introduces the possibility of sensitization (a process of becoming sensitive to the oil to such a degree that it can be dangerous to use) in anyone who uses the oxidized oil.

For oil blends, be sure to tightly cap the bottle and store it in the fridge between uses, to preserve the beneficial qualities of the blend. Keep in mind that some oils, like vetiver, will thicken when they get cold and will need to be removed from the fridge well before you want to use them. Keeping a shallow box in the bottom of your fridge allows you to organize all of your blends and access them easily.

Label Your Bottles

It is very important to clearly label all oils and oil blends. The bottles are quite small, but a standard label maker (the kind with a small keyboard) can easily print labels small enough. Label makers are available for a quite reasonable price at any office supply store. Be sure to get white tape rather than clear, as most bottles are dark in color — a white label shows up very well.

Part 2

Diffusing Essential Oils

Improving Your Health with Essential Oils

Mental and Emotional Health

Reproductive Health

Respiratory Health

Skin Health

Other Health Conditions

Addiction

Addiction is incredibly powerful — so powerful that millions of people never master it. It is complicated and devious, and just when you feel like you have found a way to overcome it, addiction will find another way to take control.

So it can only help to have as many tools as possible at hand to combat addiction. On days of weakness and temptation, the key is to find ways to avoid using. On days when the side effects of withdrawal are overwhelming, a blend that alleviates those side effects can help you maintain the strength to stay clean.

No essential oil blend can miraculously cure addiction, of course. (If you can prove me wrong, please let me know!) Still, there are several blends that may contribute to an environment that fosters strength, or determination, or simply helps you feel better.

Here you'll find a few blends that can assist you in battling addiction. Some are specific for certain addictions; others are more general.

Healing Help

Carry a small vial of a suggested oil or blend, or create a tiny container of smelling salts. Sniffing appropriate essential oils regularly can really help with cravings.

Single Oils

- Angelica
- Black pepper
- Black spruce
- Cacao
- Cinnamon
- Fennel
- Fir
- Frankincense
- Grapefruit
- Helichrysum
- Holy basil
- Lavender
- Peppermint
- Peru balsam
- Spikenard
- Sweet orange
- Tangerine
- Vanilla
- Vetiver

It helps to drink a
small glass of water
every time you have
a craving, to fulfill
your need for an oral
sensation — many
smokers find they
really miss the feel
of a cigarette in
the mouth.

Helichrysum is used in
medical aromatherapy
to address liver issues.
By speeding up the
detoxification of
nicotinoids, which are
cleared by the liver,
helichrysum essential
oil can help combat
nicotine cravings.

Smoke No More

*Smoking is one of the most difficult addictions to quit —
more challenging even than giving up heroin — so you'll
want to accept as much help as you can get while you
pursue this goal. This blend is very effective at reducing
cravings when used regularly.*

Blend

- **Helichrysum:** 3 drops
- **Black pepper:** 1 drop
- **Vetiver:** 1 drop

Diffuse

- *Smelling salts:* Sniff whenever the craving hits, and
  drink a small glass of water.

- *Nebulizing diffuser* in the place you tend to smoke.

- *Car plug-in diffuser* if you smoke in the car.

Oh My Aching Head!

*Withdrawal symptoms often include headaches, especially
when you're quitting coffee. This blend is very effective at
reducing headaches. Remember to drink water as well!*

Blend

- **Lavender:** 1 to 8 drops
- **Holy basil:** 1 drop
- **Peppermint:** 1 drop

Diffuse

- *Personal diffuser:* Carry smelling salts or an inhalation
  stick with you, to use when you feel a headache coming on.

Topical Treatment

The Oh My Aching Head! blend can be applied directly
to the temples, but it should be diluted in a base oil
(see page 198) first: 5 drops blend to 1 teaspoon (5 mL)
base oil. A roller applicator is great for this, and can
double as a personal diffuser.

Coffee or Sugar Cravings

Mmmm… coffee. The only thing that makes it even more yummy is sugar! Unfortunately, both substances can really ramp up the neurological response, leading to jitters and energy collapse a few hours later. This blend can help reduce cravings if used consistently. You might also want to try the Wake Up! blend (page 95) as a coffee replacement.

Blend

- **Black spruce or fir:** 3 drops
- **Cacao or Peru balsam:** 1 drop
- **Vetiver:** 1 drop

Diffuse

- *Terra cotta disc:* A drop or two of this blend on an unglazed medallion in a sunny window is a great way to extend its benefits throughout the day.

- *Shower:* This is a great blend to use first thing in the morning in the shower, for an energy boost.

Try an herbal coffee substitute: some people really love them and find they satisfy the desire for a dark, rich brew. Traditional substitutes use dandelion root, which has the added benefit of cleansing the liver.

Add licorice root or ground cinnamon to any tea blend for a sweet taste that may help you get over sugar cravings.

The Urge to Eat

It is important to differentiate food cravings from the desire to eat for reasons other than hunger. Food cravings can indicate a vitamin or mineral deficiency — consider having your levels checked at your next doctor's visit. But if you are eating to satisfy some unfulfilled emotional need, the blend below can help.

Blend

- **Sweet orange:** 3 to 5 drops
- **Vanilla:** 1 to 3 drops
- **Cinnamon:** 1 drop

Diffuse

- *Smelling salts:* Train your brain to feel full by sniffing this blend *only when full* for a week before using it to combat food cravings. Simply sniff immediately after eating, when you are feeling satisfied. After a week of training, sniff it when you think you want to eat, and it may help reduce cravings.

- *Heat-activated diffuser:* Use this blend in places you tend to stress-eat. For example, when I am under a deadline, I tend to eat more, so I diffuse this blend in my writing room to combat stress-eating.

You can substitute high-quality vanilla extract for the vanilla essential oil in the Urge to Eat blend.

Recovery from Alcohol Addiction

Alcohol addiction is an extremely serious issue. Please use this blend only to assist with your medical addiction program.

Blend
- **Angelica:** 1 drop
- **Black pepper:** 1 drop
- **Fennel:** 1 drop

Diffuse
- *Full-body bath:* Taking a warm (not hot!) bath with this blend can really help clear the effects of alcohol. Add a few drops to the bath *after* you get in (see page 26).

- *Nebulizing diffuser* in the room where you tend to relax in the evening.

If you are feeling overwhelmed by events in your day-to-day life, it may be tempting to give in to a craving. Bolster your resolve with the Fight That Craving! blend (page 103).

Obsessive Thinking

When you just cannot stop thinking about the object of your addiction, try this blend.

Blend
- **Frankincense:** 3 drops
- **Holy basil:** 1 drop
- **Vetiver:** 1 drop

Diffuse
- *Smelling salts:* When you recognize obsessive thinking, take several deep, slow breaths, then sniff this blend. Spend a moment in calm meditation after inhaling.

- *Fan diffuser:* As vetiver is a thicker oil, it is probably best to diffuse this one in a fan diffuser, as it may clog a nebulizing diffuser.

Vetiver is useful for connecting head to feet; that is, when you are feeling ungrounded and spacy, this oil can help bring you down to earth.

Anger Issues

In traditional Chinese medicine, anger is usually seen as a result of blocked energy. Generally speaking, feeling blocked leads to frustration; if energy flow is blocked long enough, energy builds up and can explode into anger.

Most of the essential oil blends here will help unblock the flow of energy and calm the fires before they have a chance to grow out of control. Others work by introducing delightful scents to shift your perspective. All will help reduce feelings of anger.

Smooth the Flow

If your anger response is arising from an ongoing energy obstruction, neroli will calm you, helichrysum will connect you to your resources, and pine will ground you.

Blend
- **Neroli:** 3 drops
- **Helichrysum:** 1 drop
- **Pine:** 1 drop

Diffuse
- *Nebulizing* or *fan diffuser* in an exercise room. Movement is the best thing for frustration.

- *Smelling salts:* Use as needed in smelling salts or another type of personal diffuser.

Smelling salts work as a fixative to hold the scent of essential oils, reducing their volatility.

Fire Flares

Anger sometimes manifests in outbursts that quickly rise and just as quickly dissipate. Consider this blend to stop a flare, and use it regularly to reduce the likelihood of flares occurring.

Blend
- **Bay laurel:** 3 drops
- **Lemongrass:** 3 drops
- **Cypress:** 1 to 3 drops

Diffuse
- *Nebulizing diffuser:* Use anywhere there is a likelihood of your anger being triggered.

- *Foot bath:* Cool that anger! The water in your foot bath should be room temperature to cool.

When using the Fire Flares blend in a foot bath, place a damp cloth with a drop of the blend on the back of your neck at the same time.

Vexation

When even the thought of a certain situation leads to feelings of anger, this blend will help by deprogramming the response. For the first week, sniff it at times when you are feeling balanced, then move to sniffing it whenever you encounter the source of your vexation.

Blend
- **Frankincense:** 3 drops
- **Fir:** 1 drop
- **Vetiver:** 1 drop

Diffuse
- *Smelling salts:* Carry these with you into any situation that is likely to irritate you.

- *Passive diffuser* in the space where frustration is likely to occur. For example, if there is tension at work, add a passive diffuser to your office before a meeting.

- *Car plug-in diffuser* if the source of your anger is road rage.

Frankincense is an excellent oil to consider when training the mind to break habits or learn a large volume of information quickly but well.

Angry Tummy

Nothing shuts down digestion faster than emotions, especially anger. This blend encourages the calm state necessary for optimal digestion.

Blend
- **Clary sage:** 5 drops
- **Anise:** 1 drop
- **Ylang ylang:** 1 drop

Diffuse
- *Nebulizing diffuser:* Diffuse this blend in the kitchen while you're preparing food, and in the dining area while you're eating.

- *Personal diffuser:* Sniff from a personal diffuser, such as a scent vial or inhalation stick, about 5 minutes before eating.

Acid indigestion and belching are common signs that emotion has disrupted the digestion process.

Topical Treatment

The Angry Tummy blend is actually best applied topically. One safe and effective option is to mix 1 drop of the blend into ¼ tsp (1 mL) of a base oil, such as olive oil. Apply the resulting mixture over the diaphragm, directly under the rib cage on the tummy.

Anxiety

It is safe to say that everyone suffers some anxious moments, but when does anxiety become a "problem"? My answer is, when it starts to interfere with your ability to function normally. For example, everyone feels at least a twinge of anxiety when taking a test, but if your anxiety is so great that it leads to poor performance on the test, then it has become a problem.

Another way to assess anxiety levels is to see how many systems in your body are affected by it. Obviously, someone feeling anxious will experience a sense of unease (an emotional symptom). But are you also unable to think rationally (a mental symptom)? Do you have a racing heart and clammy hands (physical symptoms)? Or all of the above?

Honestly, just reading that list could lead to anxiety! But it is important to be realistic about what sort of relief you can expect from essential oil diffusion. While the following blends have a track record of being effective against anxiety, please keep in mind that they may not work for everyone.

Single Oils

- Basil
- Bergamot
- Black spruce
- Cinnamon
- Frankincense
- Holy basil
- Lavender
- Lemon
- Lemongrass
- Marjoram
- Peppermint
- Pine
- Rose
- Rosemary
- Spikenard
- Sweet orange
- Vanilla
- Ylang ylang

A Word of Caution

If you experience increased physical stress along with anxiety, or have outright panic attacks, diffusing these blends is not likely to significantly address the problem. Other solutions should be sought out.

Vacillation between Anxiety and Resignation

So exhausting! Help balance your emotional state with this blend.

Blend 1
- **Lemongrass:** 5 to 8 drops
- **Holy basil:** 1 drop
- **Lavender:** 1 drop

Blend 2
- **Marjoram:** 5 drops
- **Bergamot:** 1 drop
- **Ylang ylang:** 1 drop

Diffuse
- *Nebulizing diffuser:* Diffuse for a few minutes first thing in the morning and last thing at night.

Lemongrass is both balancing and grounding, with the happy, uplifting note all citrus and citrus-like oils provide. Another plant to consider is melissa, also known as lemon balm. While melissa is known to effectively address anxiety, the essential oil is exorbitantly expensive. Consider drinking the tea instead, especially a tea made from fresh melissa leaves.

Social Anxiety

This blend has a good track record of helping people feel more comfortable in social settings.

Social anxiety is a very personal experience, so you may wish to experiment to find essential oils that comfort you. For many people — especially men — a combination of vanilla and cinnamon seems to work well. Adding lavender or rose to the blend is a good choice.

Blend
- **Basil:** 4 drops
- **Bergamot:** 3 drops
- **Lavender:** 1 drop

Diffuse
- *Personal diffuser:* Any easily portable personal diffuser that you can carry with you into the anxiety-causing event or situation will work well. Try a scent necklace, or smelling salts in a small vial.

- *Nebulizing diffuser:* If a personal diffuser is not an option, it may help to use this blend in a nebulizing diffuser before attending a social event.

- *Car plug-in diffuser:* Another good option is diffusing this blend in your car on the way to an event.

Mental Anxiety

When you're experiencing mental anxiety, especially the sense that you can no longer access familiar information, this blend both revives and calms. (See also "Brain Fog," page 91.)

If you do not care for one of the oils used in a particular blend, simply omit it.

Blend
- **Frankincense:** 5 to 8 drops
- **Peppermint:** 1 drop
- **Rosemary:** 1 drop

Diffuse
- *Personal diffuser* whenever you need to clear your mind.

- *Nebulizing diffuser* at the first sign of mental stress.

- *Car diffuser* if driving worsens your anxiety.

Anxiety-Induced Rootlessness

Sometimes we just want to float away from a situation that leads to anxiety. "Checking out" is one of the body's defenses against the trauma of stress. This blend will help you stay rooted in your body when it is not an option to be missing in action.

Blend

- **Pine:** 10 drops
- **Bergamot:** 2 to 4 drops
- **Sweet orange:** 2 drops

Diffuse

- *Nebulizing diffuser:* Use regularly to help reduce the likelihood of checking out.

Pine circulates energy back to the body, so it may be helpful for imbalances that leave you feeling exhausted.

Healing Help

Try adding my favorite grounding essential oil, vetiver — either alone or in combination with the Anxiety-Induced Rootlessness blend — to a warm (not hot) foot bath. Many people report that they can feel themselves "drop back down into the body" with the first whiff of this deeply earthy oil. It is quite viscous, however, so will not work in a nebulizing diffuser.

Anxiety-Induced Sleeplessness

Nothing keeps you awake like anxiety. This blend can help reduce anxious feelings and induce sleep. (See also "Sleep Issues," page 105.)

Blend

- **Sweet orange:** 10 drops
- **Lavender:** 3 drops
- **Spikenard:** 1 drop

Diffuse

- *Cotton ball* near your pillow or tucked into a corner of your pillowcase.

- *Humidifier* or *ultrasonic diffuser,* especially if dry air is contributing to your sleeplessness.

Spikenard is very useful in sleep disorders; it is one of the few oils I think of as actively sedating.

Anxiety from Emotional Upset

When an emotionally stressful situation makes you feel anxious, this blend is very uplifting. It should not be used too often, though, or it may become less useful over time.

Blend
- **Lemon:** 10 drops
- **Marjoram:** 5 drops
- **Basil:** 3 drops

Diffuse
- *Personal diffuser:* Inhale as needed from smelling salts or an inhalation stick.

In traditional Chinese medicine, anxiety is seen as a deficiency of trust in the *dao*, or the "way" one's life is unfolding. Meditation or focus on trust may help.

Brain Fog

There are times when we absolutely must be able to think and react clearly: in an emergency, for example, or when we are taking an exam. In these situations, the body's natural reaction is to produce adrenaline, which increases the blood supply to the brain, allowing more efficient cognition. Certain essential oils can also help improve blood circulation to the brain.

Digestive imbalances are a major cause of what is colloquially called "brain fog." Sometimes, simply supporting digestion can help clear the problem. Consider supplementing with digestive enzymes, or simply changing your diet to foods that are more easily digested.

Exhaustion has also been shown to reduce brain function (see box, below). It goes without saying that the best treatment for lack of sleep is sleep, but for those times when sleep is not an option and you need to think clearly, the blends here can help bridge the gap until sleep is possible. (See also "Sleep Issues," page 105.)

(See also "Sleep Issues," page 105.)

Single Oils

- Basil
- Bergamot
- Black pepper
- Cardamom
- Fennel
- Frankincense
- Lemon
- Peppermint
- Rosemary
- Vetiver

Research Roundup

A study published in *Occupational and Environmental Medicine* in 2000 found that, after 17 to 19 hours without sleep, the cognitive and motor performance of the study's 39 subjects was equivalent to or worse than their performance with a blood alcohol concentration (BAC) level of 0.05%. After longer periods without sleep, their performance reached levels equivalent to a BAC of 0.1%.

Wake Up, Brain!

This blend works by increasing circulation and waking up the senses.

Blend
- **Lemon:** 5 drops
- **Rosemary:** 5 drops
- **Peppermint:** 1 drop

Diffuse
- *Nebulizing diffuser:* Use wherever mental clarity is needed.

Be sure to cycle nebulizing diffusers off and on, as essential oils lose effectiveness if diffused for too long.

Ease the Gut to Clear the Brain

The food forms of these oils are all used to help make our meals more digestible. Smelling the oils may trigger the release of enzymes needed for digestion.

Cardamom seeds are used for digestive imbalances in many traditions.

Blend 1
- **Black pepper:** 1 drop
- **Cardamom:** 1 drop
- **Fennel:** 1 drop

Blend 2
- **Peppermint:** 5 drops
- **Basil:** 3 drops
- **Rosemary:** 1 drop

Diffuse
- *Smelling salts or inhalation stick:* Sniff the blend before eating, to help digestion.

Topical Treatment

The Ease the Gut blends are actually best applied topically. One safe and effective option is to mix the blend into a base oil, such as olive oil. Use a ratio of 2 drops blend to ¼ teaspoon (1 mL) base oil. Apply small amounts of the resulting mixture over the diaphragm, directly under the rib cage on the tummy.

Ground and Focus

When you are losing focus because you feel disconnected from your body (ungrounded), consider this blend.

Because vetiver is a thicker oil, avoid using it — or blends made with it — in a nebulizing diffuser, as it may clog the diffuser.

Blend
- **Frankincense:** 5 drops
- **Vetiver:** 3 drops
- **Bergamot:** 1 drop

Diffuse
- *Fan diffuser* as soon as you notice you feel ungrounded.
- *Foot bath:* Since the idea is to ground yourself, treat your feet to treat the rest of your body.

Depression and Bipolar Disorder

"Depression" is such an inadequate word for the myriad forms this condition takes. In my clinical practice, I have never seen two people experience depression in the same way. But, generally speaking, most people who are dealing with depression or bipolar disorder appreciate the balancing effects of an appropriate essential oil blend.

As when treating any other condition, you must choose your oils carefully, as some that are traditionally labeled "uplifting" may have the opposite effect, depending on your personal experiences with that scent. If a scent reminds you of a sad or traumatic experience, you aren't likely to find it uplifting.

Melissa (lemon balm) is probably the best-known and best-studied essential oil for depression, particularly when depression manifests as a part of bipolar disorder. But there are many other oils that can help those suffering from depression feel a bit more balanced.

A word of caution: Nearly all of the citrus oils are mood-boosting in small doses, but they can be sedating in larger amounts.

Single Oils

- Cinnamon
- Frankincense
- Ginger
- Lavender
- Lemon (or any citrus, really)
- Lemongrass
- May chang
- Melissa
- Peru balsam
- Sandalwood
- Vanilla
- Vetiver
- Ylang ylang

Lift, Ground and Center

Each of these blends contains one oil known to lift energy, one that brings you back into your body and one that centers your focus.

Blend 1
- **Frankincense or sandalwood:** 3 to 8 drops
- **Lemongrass:** 3 to 5 drops
- **Vetiver:** 1 drop

Blend 2
- **Lavender:** 1 to 3 drops
- **Ginger:** 1 drop
- **Ylang ylang:** 1 drop

Diffuse

- *Scent jewelry:* I love to use blend 1 in a wearable diffuser, as it is a light scent that most people enjoy, and is unlikely to annoy people in your immediate environment.

- *Inhalation stick:* This is a good alternative if you prefer to keep your healing scent to yourself; just take a whiff whenever you need it.

- *Terra cotta disc:* Place in a warm spot, to gently scent your space.

Just the name "frankincense" evokes a sense of ecstasy in people from many different cultures around the globe, as this oil (or the resin from which we get the oil) has been used in religious rites and spiritual practices for a very long time.

Smells Like Home

Try this blend anytime you are feeling a little homesick — when traveling, for example. Many people associate these scents with the comforts of home.

Blend
- **Cinnamon or sweet orange:** 1 drop
- **Peru balsam:** 1 drop
- **Vanilla:** 1 drop

Diffuse
- *Personal diffuser:* A scent necklace or smelling salts will allow you to carry this scent wherever you go.

You can substitute 1 drop of high-quality vanilla extract for the vanilla essential oil in the Smells Like Home blend.

Melissa Options

Although melissa (lemon balm) is known to be an effective treatment for depression, it is, unfortunately, incredibly expensive. However, if you are lucky enough to have a compounding pharmacy near you, it may be possible to obtain this oil in a dilution. Many studies have shown that this oil is actually *most* effective in a very dilute state: 1:99

Alternatively, consider growing melissa in pots placed around your house, especially near doors and windows; your heat and motion as you pass will release the scent into your house. Snipping off a few fresh leaves for a cup of tea will deliver the balancing benefits of the plant for a lot less money. Be sure to grow it in pots, though — melissa can take over a garden in no time!

Fatigue and Low Energy

There are very few people who have boundless reserves of energy, especially these days, when we are offered so many options to fill our time and wear us out. Some people find it difficult to get up in the morning, while others feel a drop in energy in the afternoon, especially after a big lunch. In addition, our penchant for traveling all over the globe has resulted in many opportunities to throw off our internal clock, disrupting our sleep and generally leading to fatigue.

Eating well, sleeping on a regular cycle, finding the time to relax during a hectic day — all of these practices will help with energy imbalances. It is not always possible to maintain a healthy routine, though. When you find yourself needing a bit more energy, consider these oils and blends. All may offer a boost when you need it most.

Single Oils

- Basil
- Bergamot
- Black pepper
- Black spruce
- Cardamom
- Carrot seed
- Cypress
- Helichrysum
- Holy basil
- Juniper berry
- Lemon
- Lemongrass
- Peppermint
- Pine
- Rose geranium
- Rosemary

Wake Up!

You may just give up coffee once you try this blend! It's very effective at getting the blood pumping in the morning.

Blend
- **Bergamot:** 3 drops
- **Black spruce:** 1 drop
- **Helichrysum:** 1 drop

Diffuse
- *Shower:* During your morning shower, add a few drops of the blend to a damp washcloth and fold the cloth so that the oils will not directly touch your skin. Lightly scrub your whole body fairly quickly, to ensure that the oils are spread evenly.

I have a dear friend who uses the Wake Up! blend in a nebulizing diffuser with a timer, set to release the scent about 1 minute before her alarm goes off. In addition to helping her awaken feeling energized, the blend usually wakes her before the strident ring, a much more peaceful way to rise!

Get Past the Midafternoon Slump

As we digest lunch, the body diverts most of its energy to the digestive system, resulting in a slump in energy a few hours later. To keep vitality high, diffuse one of these blends in your environment.

Blend 1
- **Lemon or lemongrass:** 5 to 8 drops
- **Basil:** 1 drop
- **Rosemary:** 1 drop

Blend 2
- **Peppermint:** 1 drop
- **Pine:** 1 drop
- **Rosemary:** 1 drop

Diffuse

- *Nebulizing or ultrasonic diffuser:* Make sure it's okay with everyone who shares your space before diffusing!

- *Passive diffuser:* This might be the best way to diffuse in a public work space, as passive diffusers usually scent the room just long enough to be effective without becoming overwhelming.

- *Inhalation stick:* Sniff once every 5 minutes until you feel renewed energy.

If you want to diffuse an oil in a public place, consider peppermint — I have never had a single negative response to this oil in all my years of diffusing.

Fight Jet Lag

While no essential oil has the ability to correct a confused internal clock, using these oils while you're in the air will help you arrive feeling fresh and less fatigued.

Blend
- **Cypress:** 3 drops
- **Rose geranium:** 3 drops
- **Helichrysum:** 1 drop

Diffuse

- *Spritzer:* Use a small spray bottle, so you can surreptitiously spritz your clothes while on the plane.

- *Personal diffuser:* Smelling salts work, but an inhalation stick might be more discreet.

Place 1 drop of peppermint essential oil on your fingertip as you open the air vent on the plane. This acts to both refresh your energy and help combat any microbes spread via the recirculating air.

Overcome a Hangover

This blend mostly works to help clear toxicity of the liver, but also helps settle the stomach.

Blend
- **Cardamom:** 3 drops
- **Carrot seed:** 1 drop
- **Juniper berry:** 1 drop

Diffuse
- *Shower:* Add 1 drop of the blend to a damp washcloth and fold the cloth so that the oils will not directly touch your skin. Gently scrub your upper body with the cloth, then place it over your face to breathe in the blend.

- *Nebulizing diffuser:* If you're struggling to make it as far as the shower, use a nebulizing diffuser. Plan ahead and have the blend on hand, so you can get it going easily when you first wake up.

Carrot seed has a particular affinity for the liver, and can help clear toxins.

Improve Endurance

Black spruce works like no other to get energy flowing. It does this by prompting the adrenal glands to produce more of the hormones that wake you up. Don't overdo it, or you may come to rely on it!

Blend
- **Black spruce:** 3 drops
- **Cypress:** 3 drops
- **Lemongrass:** 1 to 3 drops

Diffuse
- *Scent necklace:* This may be the best choice here, so you can have it when you find your energy flagging. Be sure to wear it only when you need it, though, so it does not stop being effective!

- *Ultrasonic diffuser* at your desk or in your work area for marathon work sessions.

- *Spritzer:* A small spritzer can be easily carried to events that will drain your energy. Add the blend to a small amount of water, and remember to shake vigorously before spritzing.

Like a breath of fresh air, the fruity sweetness of cypress can revive a dull mind.

Focused Energy

For those times when fatigue makes it difficult to get anything done, this blend helps focus your attention on the tasks at hand.

Blend
- **Holy basil:** 3 to 5 drops
- **Bergamot:** 1 drop
- **Rosemary:** 1 drop

Diffuse
- *Nebulizing diffuser* if your tasks are confined to a single room.
- *Inhalation stick:* If you're moving around to accomplish your to-do list, carry this energizing scent with you to sniff as needed.
- *Spritzer:* Add the entire blend to $\frac{1}{4}$ cup (60 mL) of distilled water for a refreshing spritz.

Citrus oils such as bergamot can be sedating in large amounts but are uplifting when used judiciously. To take advantage of the uplifting effects without getting bogged down, never use more than 5 to 8 drops at a time, and diffuse only for a few minutes at a time (10 to 15 minutes max).

Low Libido

Nothing puts a damper on a romantic evening like exhaustion, worry or stress. The best way to increase libido is to prepare! Rest before the evening starts, or take a relaxing bath (but not too hot — too much heat can be exhausting). A short meditation may help you become aware of any stress you may be unconsciously carrying. Be sure to eat moderately and avoid excess alcohol. In addition, consider diffusing essential oils to help you set the mood.

Oils you associate with a positive emotional state like joy or relaxation will be most effective. But keep in mind that certain scents that evoke positive feelings can still be a poor choice here: if the smell of roses reminds you of your grandmother, keep it out of the bedroom!

Single Oils

- Cardamom
- Cedarwood
- Cinnamon
- Clary sage
- Frankincense
- Ginger
- Grapefruit
- Jasmine
- Oakmoss
- Patchouli
- Rose
- Rose geranium
- Sandalwood
- Vanilla
- Vetiver
- Ylang ylang

Stimulating Interest

Although we like what we like, regardless of gender, over the centuries some scents have been used more for men's blends and some more for women's. Scent associations are so strong, especially over the long term, that collective memory may still play a role in what scents we find appealing, or arousing! Experiment with these oils to find what best stimulates you and your partner.

- **Male scents:** cardamom, cinnamon, oakmoss, vanilla
- **Female scents:** clary sage, jasmine, rose, rose geranium, ylang ylang
- **Neutral scents:** cedarwood, frankincense, patchouli, sandalwood

Get Comfortable

This blend is said to elicit feelings of safety and comfort, so if insecurity is getting in the way of your libido, give it a try.

Blend
- **Vanilla:** 3 drops
- **Cinnamon:** 1 drop
- **Ylang ylang:** 1 drop

Diffuse
- *Heat-activated diffuser:* Heat diffusion is nice for this blend — the resulting aroma is like the smell of baking wafting through the house.

You can substitute 1 drop of high-quality vanilla extract for the vanilla essential oil in the Get Comfortable blend.

Return to Your Body

If you become so stuck in your head or emotional state that you find it hard to feel the sensations of your body, this blend may help bring your focus back. Do be aware that it has a musky scent that some people may not enjoy, so experiment before you are in the bedroom. Be sure to blend it just before you plan to use it, so the scent is associated solely with a return to sensation (a type of entrainment).

Blend
- **Cardamom:** 3 drops
- **Vetiver:** 3 drops
- **Patchouli:** 1 drop

Diffuse
- *Heat-activated diffuser:* The heat from a candle-heated diffuser or scented wax warmer will help release the scent and set the mood.
- *Fan diffuser:* This type of diffuser is a good choice for diffusing viscous oils, such as vetiver, that could clog a nebulizing diffuser.

Oakmoss may be used in place of vetiver in the Return to Your Body blend, but keep in mind that it is very earthy — some people may find it *too* earthy.

Leave Cares Behind

The mental stressors of the day often linger long after we believe we have let them go. Euphoric oils may be just the thing to help you put them behind you.

Blend
- **Sandalwood:** 3 to 5 drops
- **Jasmine or ylang ylang:** 1 drop
- **Rose:** 1 drop

Diffuse
- *Nebulizing diffuser:* Diffuse for a few minutes at the end of the day, to help you unwind.
- *Bath salts:* Mix 3 drops of the blend into a handful of salt and add to your bath after you sit down in the tub.

Many people find rose oil to be centering, calming and uplifting, and some describe it as spiritually grounding. It is often used in libido formulas for its warming, moisturizing properties.

Stimulate!

Grapefruit is revitalizing, while both ginger and cinnamon increase blood flow and may increase sensitivity to touch.

Blend
- **Grapefruit:** 5 drops
- **Cinnamon:** 1 drop
- **Ginger:** 1 drop

Diffuse
- *Nebulizing* or *fan diffuser* in the bedroom or wherever foreplay happens!
- *Full-body bath:* Add only 1 drop of this blend, *after* getting in the water! It will spread out over the water upon contact, but even so, sitting down after adding this can burn sensitive tissues. We are trying to stimulate, not irritate, the erogenous zones!

Grapefruit oil is incredibly fresh and uplifting, without being overwhelming.

Topical Treatment

Before adding the Stimulate! blend to a diffuser, first add a few drops to the massage oil you plan to use.

Remember Pleasure

With libido, if you don't use it, you lose it. This can be a good thing or a not-so-good thing. If there is no need for it, its absence can be something of a blessing. But if the opportunity for sexual pleasure has reentered your life and your libido is MIA, consider this blend, especially alongside other techniques for waking up the body and mind.

Blend
- **Rose geranium:** 3 drops
- **Clary sage:** 1 drop
- **Jasmine:** 1 drop

Diffuse
- *Personal diffuser:* Use as needed — or desired! Try a scent necklace or an inhalation stick.

Perhaps the most intensely floral, euphoric scent known, jasmine has an extremely long history of use to enhance sexual arousal.

Topical Treatment

Add 1 drop of cinnamon essential oil (no more) to 1 tbsp (15 mL) coconut oil and apply topically to stimulate erogenous zones. *Use care!* Patch-test first on the inner thigh. And be aware that some oils can break down latex: be careful if using latex-based birth control.

Overwhelm

"Overwhelm" is an interesting word stemming from "whelm," a rarely used word that means "to be submerged." When we are so buried in tasks, thoughts, concerns or fears that we feel we cannot get out from under them, we are overwhelmed. For the most part, the solution is to retreat for a while, to rebuild our resources until we feel capable of facing the issues again. But sometimes it's just not possible for us to take the rest time we need.

The oils and blends here can help in a number of ways. They may fortify you enough to make it through another hour; they may provide clarity of thought so you can realistically assess what needs doing; or they may allow you to relax so you can build the stamina you need to face the next day.

The best course of action for you in the moment may require some thought, but these suggestions should offer some help to get you through most situations.

Single Oils

When you cannot take time to rest:

- Black pepper
- Black spruce
- Fir
- Frankincense
- Grapefruit
- Helichrysum
- Lemon
- Rosemary
- Vetiver

When you can take time to rest:

- Blue chamomile
- Clary sage
- German chamomile
- Lavender
- Rose
- Rose geranium
- Sandalwood
- Spikenard
- Sweet orange

If you are literally running a marathon, add a drop of the Finish That Marathon! blend to a tissue and tuck the tissue into a hem to smell as needed.

Finish That Marathon!

When you feel wiped out but are not quite finished with the task at hand, consider this blend.

Blend
- **Grapefruit:** 10 drops
- **Black spruce:** 5 drops
- **Black pepper:** 3 drops

Diffuse
- *Nebulizing diffuser* in your work space or wherever you need added motivation.
- *Personal diffuser:* Carry smelling salts or an inhalation stick with you to use as needed.

Ace That Exam!

This blend is particularly good to use while studying: one sniff and brain fog starts to clear.

Blend
- **Frankincense:** 5 drops
- **Lemon:** 5 drops
- **Rosemary:** 3 drops

Diffuse

- *Smelling salts:* While you're studying, occasionally sniff smelling salts infused with this blend. When it is time for the test, carry a small container of the salts with you — when you smell them, your brain will recall the information you learned while studying because it is associated with the scent! If you're worried that carrying a tin of salt into a test looks dodgy, try wearing a scent necklace instead.

Very few scents will wake up your brain the way rosemary does. Rosemary essential oil should be considered for any cognitive oil blend.

Fight That Craving!

If you are working to overcome an addiction, feeling overwhelmed may lead you to give in to your craving. Strengthen your resolve with this blend.

For more help with battling addiction, see pages 81–84.

Blend

- **Grapefruit:** 8 drops
- **Black pepper:** 5 drops
- **Helichrysum:** 3 drops

Diffuse

- *Nebulizing diffuser* in your house to keep cravings at bay.

- *Personal diffuser:* Carry an inhalation stick or smelling salts to sniff as needed.

Take Me Away …

This calming and centering blend is perfect for floral lovers. It will help you relax so you can face your to-do list the next day in a more refreshed state.

Blend

- **Sandalwood:** 3 to 5 drops
- **Lavender:** 1 drop
- **Rose:** 1 drop

Be sure to use sandalwood oil that comes from an ethically harvested source.

Diffuse

- *Full-body bath or foot bath:* Add a few drops *after* getting into the bath or submerging your feet, to really benefit from the diffusion of the scent molecules released by the warmth of the water.

Rest and Renew

Sleep does not always renew, especially if you have a lot on your mind. This blend may relax your body, to help it repair overnight.

Sweet orange oil tends to move energy up to encourage a reciprocal downward flow. The initial movement lifts us up, and the reciprocal flow helps us relax. As a result, sweet orange oil can be both uplifting and sedating, depending upon the amount used and the length of your exposure to it.

Blend
- **Sweet orange:** 3 drops
- **Black pepper:** 2 drops
- **Spikenard:** 1 drop

Diffuse
- *Nebulizing or fan diffuser:* Use anytime you have a few moments to relax and restore your energy, or in the bedroom at night. Run the diffuser for a maximum of 15 minutes while you're in the room with it, but if using it before bedtime, turn the diffuser on at least 30 minutes before you normally try to sleep, to give the sweet orange a chance to shift from stimulating to sedating.
- *Full-body bath or foot bath:* Add a few drops *after* getting into the bath or submerging your feet, to really benefit from the diffusion of the scent molecules released by the warmth of the water.

Rest and Rethink

When the brain becomes overwhelmed and needs a rest, try this blend. It will make thinking easier!

If you do not care for one of the oils used in a particular blend, simply omit it.

Blend
- **Frankincense:** 3 to 5 drops
- **Lemon:** 1 to 3 drops
- **Rosemary:** 1 drop

Diffuse
- *Heat-activated diffuser:* These scents really open up with heat.
- *Personal diffuser:* Carry or wear any of the personal diffusers to use as needed.

Sleep Issues

When bedtime has come and gone, and the whole world is asleep, why are you still awake? Or, just as frustrating, why are you waking at 2:00 a.m., unable to fall back to sleep? How can a single night seem so long?

Sleep issues are exhausting in every way. The oils and blends here are known to help address the various ways sleep can elude us. Some are calming, while some are actually sedative, but all are wonderful ways to bring on heavy lids.

Single Oils

- Frankincense
- Lavender
- Marjoram
- Red mandarin
- Roman chamomile
- Rose
- Sandalwood
- Spikenard
- Sweet orange
- Vetiver

Tips for a Good Night's Sleep

We are often our own worst enemies when it comes to establishing normal sleep cycles. In addition to diffusing essential oils to help you sleep, consider these other helpful strategies:

- Avoid screen time — television, computers, smartphones, tablets, e-readers — for at least 1 hour before bed. The light from these screens disrupts the melatonin cycles that govern sleep, and the on-screen content tends to be stimulating.

- Stop consuming stimulant foods, especially sugar, at least 1 hour before bed.

- Use only soft, warm lighting at night.

- Try to block all light from the bedroom.

- Set a regular bedtime and stick to it, even if sleep does not come right away. Rest or meditate, or visualize relaxing and falling asleep. Counting sheep does work!

- Recite affirmations to let go of stressful thoughts that may be leading to sleeplessness.

Relaxing into Sleep

This blend is very helpful for relaxing any tension in your body that is contributing to sleeplessness.

Blend

- **Lavender:** 3 drops
- **Marjoram:** 1 drop
- **Roman chamomile:** 1 drop

Diffuse

- *Humidifier:* Because tension is associated with dryness, a humidifier may be the best option here, as it delivers both warm, moist air and scent diffusion. Use at bedtime for a few minutes before you try to sleep.

- *Nebulizing diffuser:* At least 30 minutes before you plan to go to bed, diffuse this blend near you for a few minutes.

- *Full-body bath:* Taking a warm bath before bed can really help with sleep. Add a few drops of the blend to the bath *after* getting into the warm (not hot!) water, to really benefit from the diffusion of the oils.

- *Spritzer:* Spray the blend into the air in your bedroom or over your bedcovers. If spraying onto fabric, be sure to patch-test a corner first, to make sure it does not stain.

- *Cotton ball:* Add 1 or 2 drops of the blend to a cotton ball and tuck it into the corner of your pillowcase. Make sure it is at one end of the pillowcase, and not near your eyes.

Unlike its German cousin, Roman chamomile does not turn blue when steam-distilled, one of the easiest ways to ensure you are using an oil from the correct species.

Healing Help

Create a sleep pillow. It can be as simple or elaborate as you like. Make up a blend of herbs known to help with sleep, such as lavender, rose petals, mugwort, marjoram and/or melissa. Always add a small amount of hops, a known sedative herb. (Now you know why beer makes you sleepy!) Mix the herbs with rice bran hulls for a soft, light pillow, or flax seeds for a heavier pillow. Use a small cloth bag (or an altered pillowcase) to hold the mix and sew it closed. If you add essential oils to the pillow, be sure to place them in a corner, so you won't get the oils in your eyes as you sleep.

Just Knock Me Out!

Here's the most sedative blend I know!

Blend
- **Sweet orange:** 8 to 10 drops
- **Marjoram:** 3 drops
- **Spikenard:** 1 drop

Diffuse

- *Nebulizing diffuser:* At least 30 minutes before you plan to go to bed, diffuse this blend near you for a few minutes.

- *Spritzer:* Spray the blend into the air in your bedroom or over your bed covers. If spraying onto fabric, be sure to patch-test a corner first, to make sure it does not stain.

- *Cotton ball:* Add 1 or 2 drops of the blend to a cotton ball and tuck it into the corner of your pillowcase. Make sure it is at one end of the pillowcase, and not near your eyes.

> Spikenard is warming and moisturizing, and moves energy down, making it indispensable for grounding and very useful in sleep disorders. It is one of the few oils I think of as actively sedating.

What Dreams May Come

This blend encourages dreams and discourages nightmares.

Blend
- **Frankincense:** 3 drops
- **Rose:** 1 to 3 drops
- **Sandalwood:** 1 drop

Diffuse

- *Humidifier or nebulizing diffuser:* At least 30 minutes before you plan to go to bed, diffuse this blend near you for a few minutes.

- *Cotton ball:* Add 1 or 2 drops of the blend to a cotton ball and tuck it into the corner of your pillowcase. Make sure it is at one end of the pillowcase, and not near your eyes.

> Mugwort herb or essential oil has been used for centuries to encourage dreams, but some people find that it encourages very intense and vivid dreams, which may be counterproductive to sleeping through the night!

Menopause

Transitioning out of the menstrual cycle can be complicated. All women who live long enough experience this shift, but no two seem to do so in the same way. For some, the change is smooth and easy, while other women find themselves really struggling with the aftereffects of this massive hormonal shift.

Menopausal imbalances primarily involve temperature regulation, moisture regulation and emotional lability. The oils and blends here can help.

Single Oils

- Bay laurel
- Carrot seed
- Clary sage
- Cypress
- Frankincense
- Holy basil
- Lavender
- Lemongrass
- Patchouli
- Peppermint
- Rose
- Sandalwood
- Spikenard
- Sweet orange

Like lemon, lemongrass is both cooling and drying, but lemongrass acts more by dispersing fluids (rather than astringing tissues, as lemon does).

Night Sweats

Until you have awakened in a pool of sweat for the fourth time in one night to change the sheets again, it is impossible to understand how disruptive night sweats can be. This blend is cooling and drying, and will help you get a good night's sleep.

Blend
- **Lemongrass:** 3 to 5 drops
- **Bay laurel:** 1 to 3 drops
- **Peppermint:** 1 drop

Diffuse
- *Nebulizing diffuser:* Diffuse near you for a few minutes about 30 minutes before you go to bed.
- *Inhalation stick:* Keep by the bed to sniff if you awaken in the night.

Healing Help

Consider a "cool pillow." These commercial products are designed to keep the back of your neck and head cool. Because our main reserves of temperature-regulating tissue are located at the back of the neck, a cool pillow can really help keep you cool at night. To enhance the effect, spritz a little of the Night Sweats blend onto a tissue, cotton pad or cotton ball to tuck into the corner of the pillowcase.

Hot Flashes

For those waves of heat that stop you in your tracks, consider this blend.

Blend
- **Lavender:** 3 to 5 drops
- **Peppermint:** 1 to 3 drops
- **Clary sage:** 1 drop

Diffuse
- *Spritzer:* Add the entire blend to 2 to 4 tbsp (30 to 60 mL) of aloe vera juice or distilled water, shake well and spritz onto your face or body as needed.
- *Smelling salts:* Carry these with you to use as needed.

Clary sage oil is both cooling and moistening, making it perfect for hot, dry conditions. It has a marked effect on hormonal imbalances, like hot flashes.

Healing Help

Add the Hot Flashes blend to 2 tbsp (30 mL) of aloe vera juice or distilled water. Soak cotton pads in this mixture and store them in a glass storage container in the refrigerator. When it feels like a hot flash is imminent, or as soon as it starts, place the pad on the back of your neck. Make these up in bulk in advance, as they should not be reused.

A Word of Caution

Be sure to patch-test your spritz or soaked cotton pads first if you use aloe vera juice — some people are sensitive to aloe and find it drying.

Urinary Incontinence

When you're dealing with urinary incontinence, a common result of childbirth and other conditions of increased pressure, such as severe coughing, give this blend a try.

Blend
- **Cypress:** 3 to 5 drops
- **Holy basil:** 1 to 3 drops
- **Carrot seed:** 1 drop

Diffuse
- *Steaming chair:* Add 3 to 5 drops of the blend to the water in the steaming bowl and sit over it for at least 15 minutes. This can be repeated up to three times a day for up to a month. If no benefits are seen, discontinue use.
- *Shower:* Add 1 to 3 drops of the blend to a damp washcloth and fold the cloth so that the oils will not directly touch your skin. Gently press the cloth to your perineal area while you shower.

Cypress oil is cooling and moistening and can therefore be very helpful in urinary imbalances.

Vaginal Dryness

The reduction in estrogen that happens with menopause can often cause dryness. While any part of the body can experience this dryness, vaginal dryness is particularly uncomfortable. Using this blend over time can help increase secretions, lubricating and moisturizing the tissues. It works well in conjunction with the Low Libido blend, below.

Patchouli oil is warm and moisturizing, and draws energy inward to assist with repair.

Blend
- **Frankincense:** 3 drops
- **Patchouli:** 1 drop
- **Rose:** 1 drop

Diffuse
- *Steaming chair:* Add 3 to 5 drops of the blend to the water in the steaming bowl and sit over it for at least 15 minutes. This can be repeated up to three times a day for up to a month. If no benefits are seen, discontinue use.

- *Shower:* Apply a few drops to a damp washcloth and fold the cloth so that the oils will not directly touch your skin. Gently press the cloth to your mons while you shower.

Low Libido

Sadly, it is not only vaginal dryness that reduces the desire for intercourse in menopause. Libido often ebbs with the shift in hormones. This exotic, titillating blend has helped many women remember the joy of desire.

Rose oil is often used in libido blends for its warming, moisturizing properties.

Blend
- **Sandalwood:** 3 drops
- **Clary sage:** 1 drop
- **Rose:** 1 drop

Diffuse
- *Ultrasonic or nebulizing diffuser:* Diffuse near you for a few minutes about 30 minutes before you want to become intimate.

- *Scent necklace:* Wear your scent necklace as you prepare for your encounter. Your body heat will help release the scent, reminding you of what is to come.

Restless Leg Syndrome

Here's another really uncomfortable experience — and it usually starts just when sleep is nearly upon you. Be sure to diffuse this blend about 30 minutes before you settle down to sleep.

Blend

- **Lavender:** 3 to 5 drops
- **Clary sage:** 1 to 3 drops
- **Sweet orange or spikenard:** 1 drop

Diffuse

- *Nebulizing diffuser:* Diffuse near you for a few minutes about 30 minutes before you go to bed.

Topical Treatment

The Restless Leg Syndrome blend can also be added to a base oil, such as coconut oil, and applied directly to the legs. Use a ratio of 1 drop blend to ¼ teaspoon (1 mL) base oil.

Restless leg syndrome has been linked to both low magnesium (a relaxing mineral) and, oddly, low calcium, which mostly works in the body to help with contractions of all sorts. If you try one of these minerals and it does not help reduce restless leg syndrome, consider trying the other.

Menstrual Imbalances

Single Oils

- Anise
- Basil
- Bay laurel
- Carrot seed
- Clary sage
- Cypress
- Fir
- Frankincense
- Helichrysum
- Juniper berry
- Myrrh
- Patchouli
- Roman chamomile
- Rose
- Rose geranium
- Rosemary
- Tarragon
- Vetiver
- Ylang ylang

Sadly, menstrual imbalances seem to be the norm these days. Some researchers believe the culprit is our increased environmental exposure to xenoestrogens, substances that confuse the endocrine system because they are very similar to naturally occurring estrogen. Reducing your exposure to plastics and synthetic fragrances, the two worst offenders, may help regulate your cycle. We are exposed to these substances pretty much all day every day, so this is not all that easy to accomplish, but awareness is key — research alternative options to help both yourself and the planet.

In the meantime, these oils and blends can provide some relief from many common menstrual irregularities.

Cramping and Pain

If the onset of your period is associated with cramping and pain, try to use this blend every day for at least 3 days before onset — and preferably a week before — to offset the tendency.

Blend
- **Clary sage:** 3 drops
- **Roman chamomile:** 1 to 3 drops
- **Tarragon:** 1 drop

Diffuse
- *Nebulizing diffuser:* Diffuse for a few minutes at bedtime.
- *Shower:* Apply a drop or two of the blend to a damp washcloth and fold the cloth so that the oils will not directly touch your skin. Gently press the cloth to your lower abdomen for a few minutes while you shower.

Tarragon is a strongly antimicrobial essential oil and has anesthetic properties as well, making it especially useful in treating the pain of spasm.

Topical Treatment
Add the Cramping and Pain blend to a base of evening primrose oil and apply it to the lower abdomen. Use a ratio of 1 to 3 drops blend to ¼ teaspoon (1 mL) base oil.

Premenstrual Syndrome

What is premenstrual syndrome, or PMS, anyway? Every woman I know who experiences it seems to describe it differently! Regardless of how PMS manifests, this blend helps balance the head (thoughts), heart (emotions) and body. Use it for at least a week before bleeding starts, and as often as needed afterwards.

Blend
- **Frankincense:** 1 to 3 drops
- **Rose:** 1 drop
- **Vetiver:** 1 drop

Diffuse

- *Fan diffuser:* Because of the viscous vetiver, this diffuser is the best choice. Diffuse for a few minutes at bedtime.

- *Shower:* Apply a drop or two of the blend to a damp washcloth and fold the cloth so that the oils will not directly touch your skin. Gently press the cloth to your lower abdomen for a few minutes while you shower.

Many people find rose oil to be centering, calming and uplifting, and some describe it as spiritually grounding.

Topical Treatment

Add the Premenstrual Syndrome blend to a base oil, such as evening primrose oil, and apply it to the lower abdomen. Use a ratio of 1 to 3 drops blend to ¼ teaspoon (1 mL) base oil.

Irregular Schedule

*If your flow is normal but the timing of your period tends to be irregular, consider this blend. It is very important to use it regularly! Use it every day **at the same time each day**. Basically, you are trying to reset your internal clock to regulate your cycle.*

Blend
- **Rosemary:** 3 drops
- **Basil:** 1 to 3 drops
- **Anise:** 1 drop

Diffuse

- *Nebulizing or ultrasonic diffuser:* Diffuse for a few minutes at bedtime. If that is inconvenient, just be sure to use it at the same time each day.

- *Inhalation stick:* If you don't have access to a nebulizing or ultrasonic diffuser, an inhalation stick is a good option.

After your cycle is regulated, use this blend occasionally to maintain the new rhythm.

Irregular Flow

If the timing of your menstrual cycle is regular but your flow is not, consider using one of the following four blends.

Stagnant Flow

Stagnant flow manifests as very dark (purplish) blood with lots of clots. Its arrival is sometimes sudden and dramatic. You may also exhibit other signs of stagnant blood, such as spider veins or a purplish tongue. Use this blend every day for at least a week before the onset of menstruation to get your blood moving.

Blend
- **Helichrysum:** 1 to 3 drops
- **Roman chamomile:** 1 to 3 drops
- **Carrot seed:** 1 drop

Diffuse
- *Nebulizing diffuser:* Diffuse for a few minutes at bedtime.
- *Shower:* Apply a drop or two of the blend to a damp washcloth and fold the cloth so that the oils will not directly touch your skin. Gently press the cloth to your lower abdomen for a few minutes while you shower.

> **Topical Treatment**
>
> Add the Stagnant Flow blend to a base oil, such as hazelnut oil, and apply it to the lower abdomen. Use a ratio of 1 to 3 drops blend to ¼ teaspoon (1 mL) base oil.

Helichrysum oil is healing on many levels, but primarily acts to circulate energy evenly around the body. It is neither hot nor cold, and neither drying nor moisturizing, and can therefore be appropriate for a wide variety of imbalances.

Deficient Flow

Deficient blood is pale, even pinkish, and scanty. Women with deficient periods also tend to be pale and exhausted. Use this blend every day for at least a week before the onset of menstruation to build up your blood flow.

Blend
- **Juniper berry:** 3 drops
- **Myrrh:** 3 drops
- **Patchouli or rose:** 1 drop

Diffuse

- *Nebulizing diffuser:* Diffuse for up to 15 minutes at bedtime.
- *Shower:* Apply a drop or two of the blend to a damp washcloth and fold the cloth so that the oils will not directly touch your skin. Gently press the cloth to your lower abdomen for a few minutes while you shower.

Nebulizing diffusers are best used with a timer, as they are so effective it is really easy to overdo it — 10 to 15 minutes of use is usually sufficient.

Topical Treatment

Add the Deficient Flow blend to a base oil, such as rosehip oil, and apply it to the lower abdomen. Use a ratio of 1 to 3 drops blend to ¼ teaspoon (1 mL) base oil.

Dripping

This is the period that seems to never end. It can go on for a week or more and can occur more often — every three weeks, for example. There may also be spotting between cycles. The flow is never heavy, just frequent small amounts. Use this hormone-regulating blend every day until normal flow is established.

Blend
- **Cypress:** 3 drops
- **Clary sage:** 1 drop
- **Rose geranium:** 1 drop

Rose geranium oil is often used in blends to balance women's cycles.

Diffuse

- *Nebulizing diffuser:* Diffuse for a few minutes at bedtime.
- *Shower:* Apply a drop or two of the blend to a damp washcloth and fold the cloth so that the oils will not directly touch your skin. Gently press the cloth to your lower abdomen for a few minutes while you shower.

Topical Treatment

Add the Dripping blend to a base oil, such as borage oil, and apply it to the lower abdomen. Use a ratio of 1 to 3 drops blend to ¼ teaspoon (1 mL) base oil.

Flooding

This is the period that necessitates emptying the cup, changing the tampon or replacing the pad every hour or so. It may or may not be over quickly. The blood is usually bright red and does not contain many or any clots. Use this astringing blend every day for at least a week before the onset of menstruation.

Blend

- **Bay laurel:** 1 to 3 drops
- **Fir:** 1 to 3 drops
- **Ylang ylang:** 1 drop

Diffuse

- *Nebulizing diffuser:* Diffuse for a few minutes at bedtime.

- *Shower:* Apply a drop or two of the blend to a damp washcloth and fold the cloth so that the oils will not directly touch your skin. Gently press the cloth to your lower abdomen for a few minutes while you shower.

> ### Topical Treatment
>
> Add the Flooding blend to a base oil, such as hazelnut oil, and apply it to the lower abdomen. Use a ratio of 1 to 3 drops blend to ¼ teaspoon (1 mL) base oil.

If you do not care for one of the oils used in a particular blend, simply omit it.

Postpartum Vaginal Repair

Painful stretches and even tears are quite common during childbirth. In some cases, the doctor will perform an episiotomy to open space during delivery. Because the tissues around the vagina and anus have a lot of nerves, this process can be incredibly painful. Healing your injuries as quickly as possible means one less thing for you to worry about as you tend to your duties as a new mom.

These oils and blends have long been used to repair tender tissues. It is important to wait until any wounds have closed — usually 3 to 5 days after delivery — before using essential oils.

Itching

As the tissue heals, it is inevitably going to itch. Don't scratch! It can significantly delay the healing process. Soothe the itch with this blend instead.

Blend
- **Lavender:** 3 to 5 drops
- **German or blue chamomile:** 1 drop
- **Rose geranium:** 1 drop

Diffuse
- *Steaming chair:* This is an excellent way to deliver the benefits of essential oils directly to the affected area. Add 3 to 5 drops of the blend to the water in the steaming bowl and sit over it for at least 15 minutes. This can be repeated up to three times a day for up to a month. If no benefits are seen, discontinue use.

- *Sitz bath:* Use as much water as possible, remembering that much of it will be displaced when you sit down. Add 1 to 3 drops of the blend before sitting in the bath.

- *Spritzer:* Add the entire blend to a base of 2 tablespoons (30 mL) aloe vera juice or extremely diluted apple cider vinegar or witch hazel — 1 tablespoon (15 mL) ACV or witch hazel to ½ to 1 cup (125 to 250 mL) water. Shake well, then spritz onto the tender tissues as needed.

Single Oils
- Bay laurel
- Blue chamomile
- Carrot seed
- Clary sage
- Frankincense
- German chamomile
- Helichrysum
- Lavender
- Myrrh
- Peppermint
- Peru balsam
- Rose geranium
- Sage
- Sandalwood
- Thyme

Be sure to patch-test your spritz first if you choose to use aloe vera juice — some people are sensitive to aloe and find it drying.

Break Down Scar Tissue

Encourage healthy regeneration of the tissue and avoid scars in this most sensitive area. This blend encourages new healthy tissue and may reduce the likelihood of scars forming.

Blend
- **Helichrysum:** 3 drops
- **Sandalwood:** 3 drops
- **Sage:** 1 drop

Diffuse

- *Steaming chair:* Add 3 to 5 drops of the blend to the water in the steaming bowl and sit over it for at least 15 minutes. This can be repeated up to three times a day for up to a month. If no benefits are seen, discontinue use.

- *Sitz bath:* Use as much water as possible, remembering that much of it will be displaced when you sit down. Add 1 to 3 drops of the blend before sitting in the bath.

If you have access to any of the plants these oils come from, by all means use them in the sitz bath in place of the oils!

Move the Blood

The oils in this blend are known to encourage circulation, bringing immune factors to the affected area. The peppermint is also cooling.

Blend
- **Carrot seed:** 3 drops
- **Helichrysum:** 3 drops
- **Peppermint:** 1 drop

Diffuse

- *Steaming chair:* Add 3 to 5 drops of the blend to the water in the steaming bowl and sit over it for at least 15 minutes. This can be repeated up to three times a day for up to a month. If no benefits are seen, discontinue use.

- *Sitz bath:* Use as much water as possible, remembering that much of it will be displaced when you sit down. Add 1 to 3 drops of the blend before sitting in the bath.

- *Spritzer:* Add the entire blend to 2 tablespoons (30 mL) of water in the spritzer bottle (or double both amounts). Shake well, then spritz onto the tender tissues as needed.

Spritzes are best used up within a week or less, so make small amounts.

Topical Treatment

Cotton facial pads, often recommended in this book for passive diffusion (see page 21), can also be used for topical applications. Add a drop or two of the Move the Blood blend or Infected Tissue blend to aloe vera juice or cooled herbal tea, such as chamomile or peppermint. (Peppermint tea can also be used in this way on its own.) Soak a cotton pad in the mixture and apply topically.

Infected Tissue

It is quite easy for the healing tissue to become infected. These oils are strongly antimicrobial and encourage immune factors carried in the blood to move into the area.

Blend

- **Lavender:** 5 drops
- **Helichrysum:** 1 drop
- **Thyme:** 1 drop

Thyme oil has been shown to be highly effective against certain bacterial strains.

Diffuse

- *Steaming chair:* Add 3 to 5 drops of the blend to the water in the steaming bowl and sit over it for at least 15 minutes. This can be repeated up to three times a day for up to a month. If no benefits are seen, discontinue use.

- *Sitz bath:* Use as much water as possible, remembering that much of it will be displaced when you sit down. Add 1 to 3 drops of the blend before sitting in the bath.

- *Spritzer:* Add the entire blend to 2 tablespoons (30 mL) of water in the spritzer bottle (or double both amounts). Shake well, then spritz onto the tender tissues as needed.

Soothe the Pain

This blend can be used alone or added to any of the others to address the pain. Be sure to compensate for the additional oils and cut back on the amount of each blend used when diffusing.

Blend

- **Lavender:** 8 to 10 drops
- **Rose geranium:** 3 to 5 drops
- **Bay laurel:** 1 drop

Diffuse

- *Steaming chair:* Add 3 to 5 drops of the blend to the water in the steaming bowl and sit over it for at least 15 minutes. This can be repeated up to three times a day for up to a month. If no benefits are seen, discontinue use.

- *Sitz bath:* Use as much water as possible, remembering that much of it will be displaced when you sit down. Add 1 to 3 drops of the blend before sitting in the bath.

Pain is almost always accompanied by inflammation, especially at first. Bay laurel is an astringing essential oil that helps tone the boggy tissue associated with inflammation.

Prostatitis

Prostatitis and/or prostate cancer affect most men as they age. In fact, if a man lives past 80, he is almost certain to develop one or the other at some point. Fortunately, prostate cancer is so slow-growing, it is unlikely to be fatal.

Prostatitis, while also not usually fatal, can have a huge impact on quality of life. Urinary urge goes up, while urinary output goes down, meaning endless, frustrating trips to the bathroom. Any protocols that positively impact output are a sweet relief, so consider these oils and blends.

Single Oils

- Blue chamomile
- Cypress
- Ginger
- Holy basil
- Myrrh
- Oregano
- Peppermint
- Rose geranium
- Thyme

Reduced Urine Flow

This is the most common symptom men report, and the most irritating. The oils in this blend may help increase flow by reducing inflammation. They have a history of being beneficial, especially with dribbly, unsatisfying output.

Blend
- **Cypress:** 3 to 5 drops
- **Ginger:** 1 to 3 drops
- **Rose geranium:** 1 drop

Diffuse

- *Steaming chair:* This is an excellent way to deliver the benefits of essential oils directly to the affected area. Add 3 to 5 drops of the blend to the water in the steaming bowl and sit over it for at least 15 minutes. This can be repeated up to three times a day for up to a month. If no benefits are seen, discontinue use.

- *Shower:* Add a few drops of the blend to a damp washcloth and fold the cloth so that the oils will not directly touch your skin. Gently press the cloth to your perineal area while you shower.

- *Nebulizing diffuser:* Turn it on when you go to bed and set a timer to ensure that it runs for only about 15 minutes.

If you don't have a steaming chair, try sitting on a slatted stool over a steam bowl. These stools are commercially available for use in the bathroom or spa.

Blue chamomile oil is cooling to hot conditions and inflammations of all kinds.

Heat Signs

While most prostatitis manifests as "cold" — slow, dribbling, clear urine — occasionally I see a case that has "hot" symptoms: redness, heat and possibly even a burning sensation with urination. This blend will help cool the heat.

Blend
- **Holy basil:** 1 to 3 drops
- **Blue chamomile:** 1 drop
- **Peppermint:** 1 drop

Diffuse
- *Steaming chair:* Add 3 to 5 drops of the blend to the water in the steaming bowl and sit over it for at least 15 minutes. This can be repeated up to three times a day for up to a month. If no benefits are seen, discontinue use.

- *Shower:* Add a few drops of the blend to a damp washcloth and fold the cloth so that the oils will not directly touch your skin. Gently press the cloth to your perineal area while you shower.

- *Nebulizing diffuser:* Turn it on when you go to bed and set a timer to ensure that it runs for only about 15 minutes.

Infectious Prostatitis

If you observe cloudy urinary output, visit your doctor to see whether infectious prostatitis is the cause. If you are diagnosed with infectious prostatitis, this oil blend may help when used in conjunction with your doctor's other recommendations.

Both oregano and thyme are incredibly antimicrobial and have been shown to be highly effective against certain bacterial strains.

Blend
- **Cypress:** 3 to 5 drops
- **Myrrh:** 3 to 5 drops
- **Oregano or thyme:** 1 to 3 drops

Diffuse
- *Steaming chair:* Add 3 to 5 drops of the blend to the water in the steaming bowl and sit over it for at least 15 minutes. This can be repeated up to three times a day for up to a month. If no benefits are seen, discontinue use.

- *Shower:* Add a few drops of the blend to a damp washcloth and fold the cloth so that the oils will not directly touch your skin. Gently press the cloth to your perineal area while you shower.

- *Nebulizing diffuser:* Turn it on when you go to bed and set a timer to ensure that it runs for only about 15 minutes.

Vaginal Discharge

While some instances of vaginal discharge can be quite serious, for many women it is simply a rather irritating imbalance. Once your doctor has determined that the root of the issue is not a serious condition, it is easy to address discharge with essential oils. A wide variety of oils are astringing and effectively stop or slow vaginal discharge without leading to dry mucous membranes.

Soothe the Itch

If the discharge is a result of a vaginal infection, like candida, this blend has proven to be very effective.

Blend
- **Tea tree:** 1 to 3 drops
- **Rose geranium:** 1 drop
- **Rosemary:** 1 drop

Diffuse
- *Steaming chair:* Add 3 to 5 drops of the blend to the water in the steaming bowl and sit over it for at least 15 minutes. This can be repeated up to three times a day for up to a month. If no benefits are seen, discontinue use.

- *Sitz bath:* Use as much water as possible, remembering that much of it will be displaced when you sit down. Add 3 drops of the blend before sitting in the bath.

- *Shower:* Add 1 drop of the blend to a damp washcloth and apply carefully to the exterior labia. The volatile molecules of the oils are easily absorbed across the skin and may help reduce the infection.

Healing Help
The Soothe the Itch blend may also be added to yogurt thinned with water and used as a douche. Mix 1 drop of the blend into 1 cup (250 mL) of thinned yogurt and add to a douche bag.

Single Oils
- Cedarwood
- Clary sage
- Cypress
- Eucalyptus globulus
- Eucalyptus radiata
- Frankincense
- Jasmine
- Lemon
- Myrrh
- Oregano
- Patchouli
- Rose
- Rose geranium
- Rosemary
- Tea tree
- Ylang ylang

If the blend is not working as well as you would like, try eucalyptus globulus or eucalyptus radiata in place of the rosemary in the Soothe the Itch blend.

Constaflow

If the discharge is clear and copious, consider this blend.

Blend
- **Frankincense:** 3 drops
- **Patchouli:** 1 drop
- **Rosemary:** 1 drop

Diffuse
- *Steaming chair:* This is an excellent way to deliver the benefits of essential oils directly to the affected area. Add 3 to 5 drops of the blend to the water in the steaming bowl and sit over it for at least 15 minutes. This can be repeated up to three times a day for up to a month. If no benefits are seen, discontinue use.

- *Sitz bath:* Use as much water as possible, remembering that much of it will be displaced when you sit down. Add the entire blend before sitting in the bath.

If you have access to any of the plants these oils come from, by all means use them in the sitz bath in place of the oils!

Save the Undies!

If the discharge is thick and yellow, these oils may help.

Blend
- **Myrrh:** 3 drops
- **Ylang ylang:** 3 drops
- **Rose:** 1 drop

Diffuse
- *Steaming chair:* Add 3 to 5 drops of the blend to the water in the steaming bowl and sit over it for at least 15 minutes. This can be repeated up to three times a day for up to a month. If no benefits are seen, discontinue use.

- *Sitz bath:* Use as much water as possible, remembering that much of it will be displaced when you sit down. Add 3 drops of the blend before sitting in the bath.

If you don't have a steaming chair, try sitting on a slatted stool over a steam bowl. These stools are commercially available for use in the bathroom or spa.

Hormonal Shifts

If the discharge is a result of monthly hormonal shifts, try this blend.

Blend
- **Clary sage:** 1 to 3 drops
- **Rose geranium:** 1 to 3 drops
- **Jasmine:** 1 drop

Diffuse
- *Steaming chair:* Add 3 to 5 drops of the blend to the water in the steaming bowl and sit over it for at least 15 minutes. This can be repeated up to three times a day for up to a month. If no benefits are seen, discontinue use.

- *Sitz bath:* Use as much water as possible, remembering that much of it will be displaced when you sit down. Add 3 drops of the blend before sitting in the bath.

Rose geranium oil is often used in blends to balance women's cycles. Its energetic movement tends to be downward and inward — in other words, tonifying and reparative.

Lover's Leak

You may have heard of honeymoon bladder, a result of increased sexual contact. Vaginal discharge can also be triggered by a new relationship!

Blend
- **Myrrh:** 3 to 5 drops
- **Cypress:** 3 drops
- **Frankincense:** 3 drops

Diffuse
- *Steaming chair:* Add 3 to 5 drops of the blend to the water in the steaming bowl and sit over it for at least 15 minutes. This can be repeated up to three times a day for up to a month. If no benefits are seen, discontinue use.

- *Sitz bath:* Use as much water as possible, remembering that much of it will be displaced when you sit down. Add 3 drops of the blend before sitting in the bath.

- *Shower:* Add 1 drop of the blend to a damp washcloth and fold the cloth so that the oils will not directly touch your skin. Gently press the cloth to your exterior labia for a few minutes. This treatment can be repeated several times to help reduce heat and irritation.

When you're preparing a sitz bath, adding 1 to 3 drops of the blend to an emulsifying agent, such as a pinch of lecithin, can help to incorporate the oils into the water. Add the mixture to the bath after sitting, to avoid losing some of the oils' benefits to volatilization.

Allergies

When I was young, all the neighborhood kids would run around in the meadow behind our house, beating down stands of goldenrod and ragweed as we played. We did this every day, all summer long, and yet I have no memory of any of us getting itchy eyes or runny noses.

It seems pretty clear that allergic reactions and their accompanying symptoms are much more of a problem these days. The essential oils listed below may help reduce the itchy, watery eyes, runny nose and wheezing associated with allergies. See also "Rashes" (page 160) for some blends that will help with hives and other allergic rashes. And for relief from the pain of sinus congestion caused by allergies, try the Sinus Headache blend on page 165.

Constant Running

Whether it's your nose or your eyes that are running incessantly, this blend may help keep you from going mad.

Blend
- **Sandalwood:** 3 to 5 drops
- **Frankincense:** 1 drop
- **Ravintsara:** 1 drop

Diffuse
- *Shower* or *facial steamer:* If the drainage is copious and clear, try a steam. The warmth helps deliver the active compounds to where they will do the most good: into the sinuses.

- *Car plug-in diffuser:* Exposure to the outside air can make allergy symptoms worse. Use a car diffuser to nip the drip in the bud before it flowers into a full-blown attack!

Be sure to keep your eyes closed when using a facial steamer.

Stop Eye Itch!

Green myrtle, lavender, rose and quince hydrosol are all known to help soothe irritated eyes. I have sprayed all of these directly on my closed eyes with great benefit and no ill effects. Another option is to use 1 drop of blue chamomile in a facial steamer. Once the water has cooled, the remaining liquid can be used as a poultice over the eyes.

Hot and Heavy

If the discharge from your nose is thicker and associated with heat symptoms — redness, swelling, irritation — try this blend to loosen the mucus and cool the tissue.

Blend

- **Blue or German chamomile:** 3 to 5 drops
- **Inula:** 1 drop
- **Peppermint:** 1 drop

Diffuse

- *Personal diffuser:* Something more up close and personal, such as an inhalation stick or a personal nebulizing diffuser, is best for this blend.

- *Facial steamer:* The warm, moist air of a steam can really help open clogged sinuses and ease the tenderness of inflamed tissue.

Blue chamomile essential oil is bright blue and very dense; a little goes a long way. Because it is cooling, it is useful wherever there is heat, itching or irritation.

Research Roundup

A recent study found peppermint essential oil to be very effective against perennial allergic rhinitis (inflammation of the nasal passages), helping to relieve symptoms, reduce fatigue and improve quality of life.

Wheeze Squeeze

For those moments when the airways decide to spasm in response to allergens, this blend can bring some relief.

Be careful with the Wheeze Squeeze blend, as some people find it too earthy. Passive diffusion options are best.

Blend
- **Eucalyptus globulus:** 5 drops
- **Roman chamomile:** 2 drops
- **Ammi or hyssop decumbens:** 1 drop

Diffuse

- *Terra cotta disc:* Place the disc in a sunny window and let the heat of the sun diffuse the blend into the room.

- *Cotton ball:* If wheezing is keeping you awake at night, try adding a drop of the blend to a cotton ball and placing it near your bed.

Sneeze Away

This blend may help reduce the sneeze response by calming reactivity.

Unlike its German cousin, Roman chamomile does not turn blue when steam-distilled, so the color is one of the easiest ways to ensure that you are using an oil from the correct species.

Blend
- **Basil:** 1 to 3 drops
- **Roman chamomile:** 1 to 3 drops
- **Ravintsara:** 1 drop

Diffuse

- *Nebulizing diffuser* at home for a few minutes several times a day.

- *Car plug-in diffuser* when driving, to help prevent a sneeze attack in the car.

- *Personal diffuser:* Try taking a whiff from smelling salts or an inhalation stick when you're in the midst of an active sneeze attack.

Clean Out the Alley

The lymphatic system is responsible for clearing out all the detritus the body is trying to shed. If you are experiencing a constant immune reaction, the volume of detritus is enormous and the lymph can get backed up. This blend is very effective at helping the lymphatic system do the work it is supposed to do.

Blend
- **Lemon:** 3 drops
- **Bay laurel:** 1 drop
- **Ginger:** 1 drop

Diffuse
- *Facial steamer:* Steam this blend over the entire face and neck, to ensure that the lymphatic system is accessed.

- *Personal nebulizing diffuser* to focus the mist exactly where you need it.

Topical Treatment

The Clean Out the Alley blend can also be added to any base oil (see page 198) and gently smoothed over the lymph chain in the neck. Use a ratio of 3 drops blend per ¼ teaspoon (1 mL) base oil, and do not use for more than a few days.

Bay laurel oil is specific for stagnant lymph, helping to encourage circulation of the lymphatic fluid, but it is helpful for all stagnation, including respiratory fullness or stuck phlegm. It is understood to work by cooling heat and encouraging the moistening of thickened fluids.

Asthma

It is imperative that essential oils be introduced very carefully to anyone with respiratory issues (see box, below). As you might expect, strong scents can exacerbate breathing problems. Having said that, essential oils can be powerful allies in most respiratory conditions, including asthma. Some oils (such as ammi and hyssop decumbens) help with constriction, while others work to break down mucus or help move it out of the respiratory system. In addition, several of the oils listed here (ammi and frankincense, for example) may help to reduce reactive airways over time.

A Word of Caution

Never expose anyone with a respiratory condition to full-strength essential oils. Introduce oils very carefully. One way to do this is to open a bottle very quickly about 3 feet (1 m) from the person's nose (about as far as their arm's reach). If they are sensitive to the oil, this will cause a slight response — enough to demonstrate that they should not use that oil.

Thick Goo Be Gone!

This blend works wonders when you are experiencing that irritating condition of being congested but having an unproductive cough.

Blend

- **Eucalyptus globulus:** 5 drops
- **Pine:** 5 drops
- **Inula:** 1 drop

Diffuse

- *Facial steamer:* This method will effectively deliver the blend exactly where it needs to go. Add 1 to 3 drops of the blend, depending on the size of your steamer's well.

- *Shower:* Add a drop of the blend to a washcloth and place it over your face, breathing gently through your nose. Sniff the washcloth before placing it over your face to make sure the blend is not too strong or irritating.

- *Inhalation stick:* Use as often as needed to help open the passages and move thick goo.

Inula essential oil is a fantastic mucolytic, meaning it breaks down mucus. In addition, it reduces bronchospasms. Together, these two properties make inula incredibly effective against most respiratory imbalances.

Thin Goo Be Gone!

This one is better for a constant drip, postnasal or otherwise.

Blend
- **Ginger:** 3 drops
- **Eucalyptus globulus or radiata:** 1 to 3 drops
- **Peppermint:** 1 drop

Diffuse
- *Facial steamer:* This method will effectively deliver the blend exactly where it needs to go. Add 1 to 3 drops of the blend, depending on the size of your steamer's well.

- *Shower:* Add a drop of the blend to a washcloth and place it over your face, breathing gently through your nose.

- *Inhalation stick:* Use as often as needed to help open the passages and move thin goo.

Be sure to keep your eyes closed when using a facial steamer.

Loosen the Band

Try this blend to loosen the constriction felt during an asthma attack.

Blend
- **Hyssop decumbens:** 3 drops
- **Fennel:** 1 drop
- **Roman chamomile:** 1 drop

Diffuse
- *Nebulizing diffuser:* Diffuse as needed for 5 to 10 minutes at a time.

- *Smelling salts:* These may be particularly appropriate here, as there is some research that suggests the negative ions from salt may help with asthma (see Research Roundup, page 132).

Hyssop decumbens helps to open bronchial tubes very effectively, without being aggressive.

Topical Treatment

If the asthmatic spasm comes on with exercise, the Loosen the Band blend can be diluted in a base oil, such as olive or sweet almond oil, at a ratio of 5 drops blend to 1/2 teaspoon (2 mL) base oil and massaged over the diaphragm, directly under the rib cage on the tummy, before and after exercise.

Ward It Off

You may be able to prevent an asthma attack by carefully using this blend before an activity that typically brings one on.

Blend
- **Hyssop decumbens:** 1 drop
- **Fennel:** 1 drop
- **Fir:** 1 drop

Diffuse
- *Smelling salts:* Be sure to test this blend when breathing is normal before relying on it during an asthma attack.
- *Warm steam* if the air is dry. *Always* use warm, not hot, water, as excess heat can exacerbate asthma symptoms.

Hyssopus officinalis var. *decumbens* is the only hyssop variety that is appropriate for use in its essential oil form. Never use *Hyssopus officinalis* as an essential oil.

Research Roundup

A 1995 study in the *Journal of Aerosol Medicine* examined the effects on patients with various respiratory conditions of an aerosol designed to simulate the effects of the air in a natural salt cave. This approach, called halotherapy, was successful at reducing symptoms in the majority of the patients in as few as three to five sessions.

Reprogram the Reaction

If used regularly, this blend may help to reduce the reactivity of your airways over time.

Blend
- **Frankincense:** 3 to 5 drops
- **Ammi:** 1 drop
- **Cypress:** 1 drop

Diffuse
- *Terra cotta disc* set in a warm spot, like a sunny window.

Frankincense is an excellent addition to a blend when you're attempting to reprogram your body or mind.

A Word of Caution

This blend has a very strong scent that some people dislike, and it absolutely must be tested before use, as it could trigger a reaction.

Coughs

A cough can be a symptom of any respiratory condition — asthma, allergies, viral infections and so on. Physiologically, it can be described as a reflexive response to irritation in the respiratory tract. Some coughs are necessary to keep the airways clear, as when we accidentally inhale a foreign substance, but occasionally a cough is just irritating and unproductive.

Essential oils have been shown to be an incredibly effective treatment for coughs. Chest balms sold in pharmacies all over the world use essential oils (or synthetic versions of essential oils) as their active ingredients.

Some of the blends below help stop a cough, while others work to make a cough more productive, so regardless of what type of cough you are experiencing, you'll find relief here.

Topical Treatment

All of the cough blends have been designed for use in a diffuser, but they can also be added to a base oil, such as coconut oil, and applied to the chest, if preferred. Use a ratio of 5 drops blend per ¼ teaspoon (1 mL) base oil. Proceed with caution, as all strong scents can initially worsen a cough.

Single Oils

- Black spruce
- Cedarwood
- Cypress
- Eucalyptus citriodora
- Eucalyptus globulus
- Eucalyptus radiata
- Frankincense
- Hyssop decumbens
- Inula
- Lemon
- Peppermint
- Ravintsara
- Roman chamomile
- Rosemary
- Sandalwood
- Thyme

Increase Productivity

This blend can really help when your congestion is thick and you are having difficulty clearing it (expectorating).

Blend

- **Eucalyptus globulus or radiata:** 8 to 10 drops
- **Frankincense:** 3 drops
- **Inula:** 1 drop

Diffuse

- *Personal diffuser:* Inhale from a personal nebulizing diffuser or an inhalation stick as needed.

- *Facial steamer:* This method will effectively deliver the blend exactly where it needs to go. Add 1 to 3 drops of the blend, depending on the size of your steamer's well.

I have found the Increase Productivity blend to be particularly useful for excess mucus that lingers even after recovery from a cold or flu.

A Word of Caution

The Increase Productivity blend can be used frequently, but discontinue use if there is no improvement, as inula should not be used long term.

Cough with Sore Throat

Coughing when your throat is raw is just no fun at all. This blend helps soothe the throat so coughing is less painful.

Try adding 1 drop of the Cough with Sore Throat blend to 1 teaspoon (5 mL) honey. Spoon it in your mouth and let it slowly trickle down your throat to reduce viral load, soreness and irritation.

Blend
- **Eucalyptus globulus or radiata:** 5 to 8 drops
- **Ravintsara:** 5 drops
- **Lemon:** 3 drops

Diffuse
- *Personal diffuser:* Inhale from a personal nebulizing diffuser or inhalation stick as needed.

Cough Due to Chest Infection

This strongly antimicrobial blend is a good choice if there is any likelihood of infection.

Thyme is incredibly antimicrobial and has been shown to be highly effective against certain bacterial strains.

Blend
- **Eucalyptus globulus or radiata:** 3 to 5 drops
- **Frankincense:** 3 drops
- **Thyme:** 1 drop

Diffuse
- *Personal diffuser:* Inhale from a personal nebulizing diffuser or inhalation stick as needed to help reduce coughing.

A Word of Caution

The Cough Due to Chest Infection blend is particularly strong, so use it carefully. If you have any tightness in your chest, be sure to introduce it slowly and stop using it immediately if it worsens the situation.

Cough Due to Constriction

If the respiratory tract becomes constricted, the body will automatically cough in an attempt to open things up. This blend opens your respiratory tract so you can stop coughing.

Blend
- **Hyssop decumbens:** 3 to 5 drops
- **Roman chamomile:** 3 to 5 drops
- **Rosemary:** 3 to 5 drops

Diffuse
- *Personal diffuser:* Inhale from a personal nebulizing diffuser or inhalation stick as needed.
- *Facial steamer:* This method will effectively deliver the blend exactly where it needs to go. Add 1 to 3 drops of the blend, depending on the size of your steamer's well.

Hyssopus officinalis var. decumbens is the only hyssop variety that is appropriate for use in its essential oil form. Never use Hyssopus officinalis as an essential oil.

Cough Due to Postnasal Drip

These oils are known to be drying and may help reduce the constant drain of postnasal drip.

Blend
- **Eucalyptus citriodora or radiata:** 5 to 8 drops
- **Lemon:** 3 to 5 drops
- **Peppermint:** 1 to 3 drops

Diffuse
- *Inhalation stick:* This blend definitely works best if you inhale it directly into the nose, where it can do its best work.
- *Warm steam:* This option may seem counterintuitive, but the warm, moist steam will help the scent molecules get into the areas where they need to do their work.

All of the eucalyptus oils are warming and drying, perfect for damp, cold conditions like postnasal drip.

Healing Help

Adding a drop of clove oil to any of the cough blends may help reduce the pain that results from extended coughing. Clove is *intense*, so take it slow if you choose to add this powerful aid — start sniffing from arm's length away to ensure your body will tolerate the scent.

Cough Due to Overexertion

The cough reflex can be triggered by the failure to breathe deeply. In much the same way as a yawn forces us to take in a deep gulp of air, a cough can generate the physiological effect of deeper breathing.

Of course, what you really need here is rest! But when that is not possible, this blend can help. These oils are known to open the lungs and deepen the breath. They also increase stamina, so you can finish a marathon or get through an all-night study session.

Blend
- **Cypress:** 3 drops
- **Black spruce:** 1 to 3 drops
- **Cedarwood:** 1 drop

Diffuse
- *Personal diffuser:* Carry an inhalation stick or smelling salts with you to use as needed or, better yet, wear a scent necklace when exerting yourself.

- *Cotton ball:* Add a drop of the blend and place the cotton ball in a small muslin bag (to protect your clothes and skin), then tuck it into a bra or cuff.

Sinus Pain

Sinus fullness alone is enough to cause really uncomfortable pressure and pain. The lack of drainage often results in sinus infections, too. Because of the nature of sinus cavities, once an infection has gotten in, it can be terribly difficult to completely eradicate. Regular treatments with essential oils can go a long way toward keeping the sinus cavities healthy.

Healing Help

In addition to diffusing essential oils to treat your sinus pain, you may want to try a sinus irrigation technique, such as a neti pot or sinus lavage tool. A neti pot is a little pot with a spout that allows you to pour warm salty water through your nasal passages to flush out mucus. The lavage tool is a syringe or bulb that allows you to ease the sinuses open with a small amount of water pressure.

Single Oils

- Basil
- Bay laurel
- Blue chamomile
- Eucalyptus citriodora
- Eucalyptus globulus
- Eucalyptus radiata
- Helichrysum
- Lemon
- Peppermint
- Rosemary
- Thyme

Recurring Sinus Infection

Those who are prone to seemingly constant sinus infections can both prevent them and address an existing infection by diffusing this blend.

Blend
- **Eucalyptus (any type):** 1 drop
- **Peppermint:** 1 drop
- **Thyme:** 1 drop

Diffuse
- *Nebulizing diffuser* at home for a few minutes several times a day.

- *Personal diffuser:* Breathe deep from a personal diffuser, such as an inhalation stick, several times a day as needed.

- *Warm steam:* For really intransigent sinus infections, use steam liberally and often to help the scent molecules work their way into the sinus cavities.

Thyme has been shown to be highly effective against certain bacterial strains. It can be harsh and irritating, so it is best used in tiny amounts.

Hot, Inflamed Sinuses

This blend helps cool and move stagnant blood, which in turn may stimulate sinus drainage.

Blend
- **Blue chamomile:** 3 drops
- **Helichrysum:** 3 drops
- **Peppermint:** 1 drop

Diffuse
- *Nebulizing diffuser* at home for a few minutes several times a day.
- *Inhalation stick* to deliver this blend on demand, right where it needs to be.

Do not use the Hot, Inflamed Sinuses blend in a steam, as that will negate the cooling benefits it offers.

Stagnant Sinuses

When the heat of infection is absent, and you're dealing only with sluggish tissues, this blend is a better choice.

Blend
- **Rosemary:** 3 drops
- **Peppermint:** 1 drop
- **Thyme:** 1 drop

Diffuse
- *Nebulizing* or *ultrasonic diffuser* at home for a few minutes several times a day.
- *Personal diffuser:* Smelling salts may be appropriate here, to stimulate drainage.

Peppermint is both cold and hot, making it very effective at circulating energy. It is also somewhat drying, making it helpful for reducing boggy inflammation.

Lymph Drainage

Sometimes the problem is not actually the sinuses, but a lack of lymph movement. Many waste fluids are removed through the action of the lymphatic system. If lymph stagnates, other fluids have nowhere to go. Treating the lymphatic system with this blend can really help!

Blend

- **Lemon:** 3 drops
- **Basil:** 1 to 3 drops
- **Bay laurel:** 1 to 3 drops

Diffuse

- *Nebulizing diffuser* at home for a few minutes several times a day.

- *Warm steam:* Use steam liberally and often to help the scent molecules get the lymph moving. Shower steams may be best, to include all lymph chains in the body.

Bay laurel is specific for stagnant lymph, helping to encourage circulation of the lymphatic fluid. It is understood to work by cooling heat and encouraging the moistening of thickened fluids.

Dry Skin Brushing

The Lymph Drainage blend is a great one to use with dry skin brushing. This amazingly effective technique encourages movement through the lymphatic system, to keep it healthy. Lymph fluid moves just under the surface of the skin, carrying dead bacteria, white blood cells and other detritus out of the body. Like the venous system, it is primarily activated by movement — muscle contractions massage the lymph vessels and keep the system moving.

When we are sick, the lymph tends to stagnate, but we can stimulate it with dry skin brushing, which works in a similar way to muscle contractions. Dry skin brushing involves gently sweeping a dry brush with short, stiff bristles along the body, always moving in the direction of the heart. *Gently* is the key! If the brush is applied too vigorously, it bypasses the lymph and works directly on deeper structures.

To use this technique with the Lymph Drainage blend, add a few drops of the undiluted blend to your palm, vigorously rub your hands together and then quickly swipe your hands over your entire body, from your extremities in toward your central torso. Immediately follow with the dry skin brushing technique. Do this every day for 2 weeks (no longer) during cold and flu season to avoid becoming sick.

Sore Throat

A sore throat often signals the onset of a cold or flu, as it is one of their most common initial symptoms. Sore throats can also be the result of overuse after a sporting event, a rock concert or extended public speaking. Exposure to irritants is another common cause — substances such as pollen, chemical fumes and smoke can quickly lead to irritated tissues in the throat.

Whatever the cause, the pain and irritation of a sore throat are difficult to overlook, as we use our throats every second of the day, to breathe, swallow, eat and talk. These oils have a proven track record for reducing the pain and discomfort of a sore throat.

Healing Help

In addition to diffusing essential oils, try gargling with salt water (see box, page 142) and/or letting honey trickle down your throat, both of which are remedies that are known to be effective for combating the pain of sore throats.

Ravintsara essential oil is a fantastic champion against the viruses that cause sore throats. I often recommend adding 1 drop of the oil to 1 teaspoon (5 mL) honey, preferably manuka honey. Hold the mixture in your mouth and let it slowly trickle down your throat. This remedy can be used as both a preventive and to combat an existing sore throat.

Infected Throat

This blend may help fight off the infection that's causing the problem.

Blend

- **Ravintsara:** 1 to 3 drops
- **Clove or juniper berry:** 1 drop
- **Thyme:** 1 drop

Diffuse

- *Personal nebulizing diffuser:* Be warned: this blend is very strong! Do not breathe it into your lungs; rather, let the mist enter your mouth and throat passively while breathing through your nose.

- *Inhalation stick:* For this more passive diffusion method, you can breathe in gently through your mouth instead of your nose.

- *Facial steamer:* Use lukewarm water and breathe in cautiously, as always.

Soothe the Pain

When it hurts to swallow, so many other actions become more difficult! Eating, drinking, speaking, coughing and sneezing can all aggravate a sore throat. Try this blend to help ease the pain.

Blend

- **Eucalyptus (any type):** 1 to 3 drops
- **Lavender:** 1 drop
- **Ravintsara:** 1 drop

Diffuse

- *Facial steamer:* This is the best way to use this blend, as the warm, moist air is delivered exactly where it needs to go to soothe the irritated tissues. As with any steam, be very careful to use warm, not hot, water.

- *Shower:* Add a drop of the blend to a washcloth, place the cloth over your mouth and gently breathe in the scent. This has the same effect as a facial steam and is a bit easier to do if you need a shower anyway.

- *Personal nebulizing diffuser:* When the aerosol hits your throat, try to avoid breathing it into your lungs; instead, just let the oils coat your throat.

If a sore throat is making the rounds of everyone at your home or office, consider adding juniper berry to any of the blends. Herbal doctors often bite down on a juniper berry before entering a sick room, as its volatile compounds are so good at neutralizing airborne infectious agents.

Regain Your Voice

Losing your voice can make all of your daily activities more challenging. Think about how often you use your voice over the course of a day! This blend can help relax and tone irritated vocal cords.

Blend

- **Ginger:** 3 drops
- **Cinnamon:** 1 drop
- **Clove:** 1 drop

Diffuse

- *Facial steamer:* Allow the steam to gently coat your throat by opening your mouth but breathing through your nose. This is a *very* strong blend, so use caution and try not to breathe through your mouth.

The Regain Your Voice blend also works really well as a tea, using the herbs themselves!

Recover from Overuse

When it comes to relieving the raw, inflamed tissues caused by overuse, soothing, moistening oils are best.

Blend
- **Juniper berry:** 1 drop
- **Lavender:** 1 drop
- **Myrrh:** 1 drop

Diffuse
- *Nebulizing, ultrasonic or fan diffuser:* Any diffuser that does not rely on heat is a good option here. As with the other blends, allow the volatile compounds to coat your throat, rather than breathing them into your lungs.

- *Personal diffuser:* Regular gentle inhalation of this blend may be the best way to reap its benefits.

The Recover from Overuse blend is another great addition to a salt-water gargle (see box).

Salt-Water Gargle

To make a salt-water gargle, add 4 drops of either of the blends below to 1 cup (250 mL) warm water mixed with ¼ teaspoon (1 mL) salt. Try to use it up within a couple of hours — gargle ¼ cup (60 mL) once every half-hour, for example.

Blend 1
- Eucalyptus (any type): 1 drop
- Grapefruit: 1 drop
- Thyme: 1 drop

Blend 2
- Lemon: 1 to 3 drops
- Clove: 1 drop
- Myrrh: 1 drop

Try diffusing these blends in a nebulizing diffuser in addition to gargling.

Stuffy Nose

A stuffy nose is often a symptom of a deeper issue, like a sinus infection or allergies. The oils listed here have proven to be very helpful at relieving the discomfort of a stuffy nose. Most of them open the sinus passages, while others loosen thickened mucus so it can drain. Keep in mind, though, that you must address the root cause to permanently clear the symptom (see Allergies, page 126, and Sinus Pain, page 137).

(see Allergies, page 126, and Sinus Pain, page 137)

Single Oils

- Bay laurel
- Blue chamomile
- Carrot seed
- Eucalyptus citriodora
- Eucalyptus globulus
- Eucalyptus radiata
- Juniper berry
- Lemon
- Oregano
- Peppermint
- Roman chamomile
- Rosemary
- Thyme

Moisten the Dryness

Often the nose feels stuffy because the mucous membranes have dried out. The following blend is moisturizing, especially if you use steam to diffuse it.

Blend
- **Carrot seed:** 1 drop
- **Juniper berry:** 1 drop
- **Roman chamomile:** 1 drop

Diffuse

- *Facial steamer:* This method will effectively deliver the blend exactly where it needs to go. As always, be sure to keep your eyes closed when using a facial steamer.

- *Shower:* Add a drop of the blend to a washcloth and place it over your face, breathing gently through your nose.

- *Humidifier:* Running a humidifier with this blend in the bedroom while you sleep can help you heal overnight.

Juniper berry essential oil is warming, but unlike many warming oils, it is also moisturizing. It achieves its moisturizing effect primarily by redistributing fluids.

Slow the Flow!

Sometimes a stuffy nose means a constant drip! This blend is astringent without being too drying.

Blend
- **Eucalyptus (any type):** 3 drops
- **Bay laurel:** 1 drop
- **Lemon:** 1 drop

Diffuse

- *Personal diffuser:* Use an inhalation stick or smelling salts as needed.

- *Personal nebulizing diffuser:* Direct the mist from the diffuser toward the nose.

All of the eucalyptus oils are warming and drying, perfect for damp, cold conditions like a stuffy nose.

Open the Passages

This blend is fantastic when it feels like no air whatsoever is making its way through your nose.

Blend
- **Eucalyptus (any type):** 3 drops
- **Rosemary:** 3 drops
- **Peppermint:** 1 drop

Diffuse
- *Warm steam:* The warm, moist air really helps deliver the blend into the sinus cavities.

- *Inhalation stick:* Direct the essential oil molecules exactly where they need to go by inhaling as needed. Smelling salts also work, if you prefer.

Clear an Infection

This super-strong formula has a scent most people find a bit harsh, but it is incredibly effective against both viruses and bacteria. Use it carefully, especially at the beginning.

Both thyme and oregano are incredibly antimicrobial and have been shown to be highly effective against certain bacterial strains.

Blend
- **Eucalyptus (any type):** 3 drops
- **Peppermint or oregano:** 1 drop
- **Thyme:** 1 drop

Diffuse
- *Warm steam:* The warm, moist air will help open the passages and deliver the blend deep into the nasal cavities.

- *Humidifier:* Diffuse this blend while you sleep, when the body is in repair mode.

- *Inhalation stick:* If you feel you need more frequent clearing action, carry your treatment with you!

Topical Treatment

The Clear an Infection blend can be added to any base oil (see page 198) and applied topically inside the nose. Start with a tiny amount, keeping in mind that you may find the scent disagreeable: try 1 drop of the blend per ¼ teaspoon (1 mL) base oil. Use a cotton bud to dab the mixture inside your nose, but be very careful not to probe too deep, or you may damage sensitive nasal tissue.

Reduce Reactivity

If you reduce the sensitivity of your immune system, your entire body will respond with greater balance, meaning your nose is more likely to stay clear. Use this blend several times a day while retraining your immune system.

Blend
- **Blue chamomile:** 3 drops
- **Peppermint:** 1 drop
- **Roman chamomile:** 1 drop

Diffuse
- *Nebulizing diffuser:* Diffuse for 5 to 10 minutes first thing in the morning.

- *Warm steam:* If you experience near-constant drainage of clear mucus from your nose, steam may be the best way to reduce your reactivity.

- *Inhalation stick:* Use whenever you feel an allergy attack coming on.

Blue chamomile oil is very dense — a little goes a very long way. It is cooling to hot conditions and inflammations of all kinds.

Drain the Lymph

Occasionally, the nose gets stuffed up because the lymphatic system is not functioning properly. Moving the lymph may help drain the nasal passages.

Blend
- **Juniper berry:** 3 drops
- **Bay laurel:** 1 drop
- **Lemon:** 1 drop

Diffuse
- *Nebulizing diffuser:* Use at night for about 10 minutes to help the lymphatic system recalibrate.

- *Shower:* Add a drop of the blend to a washcloth and fold the cloth so that the oils will not touch your skin. *Very* gently stroke the cloth down both sides of your neck. Finish by placing the cloth over your nose and breathing in gently through the nose.

Bay laurel is specific for stagnant lymph, helping to encourage circulation of the lymphatic fluid. It is understood to work by cooling heat and encouraging the moistening of thickened fluids.

Acne

Single Oils

- **Blue chamomile**
- **Carrot seed**
- **Clary sage**
- **Eucalyptus citriodora**
- **Frankincense**
- **Helichrysum**
- **Lavender**
- **Lemon**
- **Patchouli**
- **Rose geranium**
- **Sage**
- **Sandalwood**
- **Tea tree**

No matter where they pop up, pimples are a pain, and acne is always unwelcome — not to mention that it always seems to flare up at the worst possible moment! And then there's the unpleasant reality that any attempts to treat a spot are apt to make it worse. That's where diffusion comes in: the gentle application by steam or air delivers essential oil molecules in small amounts just where they are needed, without exacerbating an already unpleasant situation.

Skin-Care Tips

- Avoid soap-based cleansers that upset the acid mantle of the skin; instead, use coconut oil! Coconut oil pulls away the grime without disrupting the acid mantle, making it a great safe cleanser.

- Acne-prone skin responds very well to diluted apple cider vinegar. For a safe facial wash, add 1 part apple cider vinegar to 9 parts water. If the vinegar is not diluted, its acidity can burn the skin.

- Aloe vera gel or juice is a great base for toners and washes, but patch-test first! Some people are sensitive to aloe and find it drying.

- Some people find baking soda effective as a spot treatment, but be warned that it is somewhat harsh.

- Hormonal acne may improve if you drink red clover tea daily, as red clover is an herb known to help with hormonal balance.

- If you are prone to acne, consider using skin-care products that contain jojoba oil, tamanu oil or apricot seed oil.

Hot Red Acne

Pimples can be very hot and painful. This blend cools and reduces the pain, while also reducing bacterial load.

Blend
- **Lavender:** 5 to 8 drops
- **Rose geranium:** 3 to 5 drops
- **Blue chamomile:** 1 to 3 drops

Diffuse
- *Spritzer:* Add the entire blend to ¼ cup (60 mL) of water or aloe vera juice. Shake well, then spritz your face or other affected body parts as needed. You can store the spritzer in the fridge for even more cooling power.

Be sure to patch-test your spritz first if you choose to use aloe vera juice — some people are sensitive to aloe and find it drying.

Cystic Acne

This painful condition responds beautifully to the use of essential oils, as they may help unclog pores and soften sebum plugs. The Cystic Acne blend also moves blood and breaks down scar tissue.

Blend
- **Tea tree:** 5 to 8 drops
- **Helichrysum:** 1 to 3 drops
- **Sage:** 1 drop

Diffuse
- *Ultrasonic diffuser:* Direct the mist toward your face or other affected body parts for several minutes several times a day.

- *Facial steamer:* For cystic acne, set your facial steamer to its coolest temperature. Add 1 to 3 drops of the blend to the steamer, depending on its size (follow the directions that accompany your steamer).

Clogged pores are part of the reason cystic acne develops. Jojoba oil is very similar in composition to the sebum produced by the skin. As counterintuitive as it seems, using jojoba oil on the areas where blackheads occur may help unclog the pores.

Topical Treatment

This blend can also be applied directly to cysts: dab it on very carefully with a cotton bud. If you find it further irritates your skin, replace the sage with 3 drops of lavender.

Infected Acne

Picking at pimples can often lead to them becoming infected, as our fingers harbor large amounts of bacteria. Picking also irritates the tissue and leads to a greater likelihood of scarring. But if you give in to the temptation to pick and infection arises, use this blend to treat it.

Blend
- **Eucalyptus citriodora:** 3 to 5 drops
- **Tea tree:** 3 to 5 drops
- **Lemon:** 1 to 3 drops

Diffuse
- *Facial steamer:* Add 1 to 3 drops of the blend to the steamer, depending on its size (follow the directions that accompany your steamer).

When using a facial steamer, remember that it is very important to keep your eyes closed throughout.

Topical Treatment

The Infected Acne blend can also be used as a spot application, but be sure to limit it to just the area of the spot. Honey, especially manuka honey, is a great base for a spot treatment. Use a ratio of 1 drop blend to 1/4 teaspoon (1 mL) honey and apply several times a day.

Acne with Blackheads

Consider this blend if your acne is accompanied by comedones (commonly called blackheads).

Blend
- **Lavender:** 3 to 5 drops
- **Sandalwood:** 1 to 3 drops
- **Tea tree:** 1 drop

Diffuse
- *Facial steamer:* Add 1 to 3 drops of the blend to the steamer, depending on its size (follow the directions that accompany your steamer).

Tea tree oil is strongly antimicrobial and healing, a perfect combination for treating acne.

Topical Treatment

A drop of the Acne with Blackheads blend can be added to an egg white or 1/4 cup (60 mL) of full-fat yogurt (but not both at the same time!) and applied over the entire face.

Hormonal Acne

Some of us get breakouts only during hormonal shifts. This blend may help balance your hormones.

Blend
- **Carrot seed:** 3 to 5 drops
- **Clary sage:** 3 to 5 drops
- **Frankincense:** 1 to 3 drops

Diffuse
- *Facial steamer:* Add 1 to 3 drops of the blend to the steamer, depending on its size (follow the directions that accompany your steamer).

Clary sage effectively helps balance hormone levels, and carrot seed is excellent at moving the blood.

Topical Treatment

Make a facial wash by adding a drop of the Hormonal Acne blend to ¼ teaspoon (1 mL) of aloe vera juice — or to warm water if you are sensitive to aloe. Rinse well. This blend is also very effective on its own as a spot treatment.

Aging Skin

As we age, our skin changes. Although skin generates growth hormone, which is responsible for tissue repair, the amount it creates often drops as we age. The skin's ability to repair itself slows, and we see the results as less tone to the tissue, slackened areas and wrinkles. (Wrinkles are a lot like scars: the tissue beneath has been so overworked that it is unable to effectively repair itself.)

Essential oils have a fantastic track record when it comes to repairing and rejuvenating skin.

Single Oils

- Blue chamomile
- Carrot seed
- Clary sage
- Frankincense
- Helichrysum
- Lavender
- Patchouli
- Rose
- Rose geranium
- Sandalwood

Sluggish Circulation

Sluggish circulation is usually accompanied by a dull pallor or by areas of darkness. Occasionally, the darkness may appear slightly purplish.

Blend
- **Rose:** 1 to 3 drops
- **Carrot seed:** 1 drop
- **Helichrysum:** 1 drop

Diffuse
- *Shower:* Add a drop of the blend to a damp washcloth and fold the cloth so that the oils will not directly touch your skin. Gently press the cloth to your face for a few minutes while you shower.

- *Facial steamer:* Add 1 to 3 drops of the blend to the steamer, depending on its size (follow the directions that accompany your steamer).

Follow your shower or facial steam by splashing your skin with cool water and giving yourself a gentle facial massage.

Liver Spots

These dark spots or patches usually occur in areas that have been repeatedly exposed to the sun, like the face or hands. They are very common in people over the age of 50.

Blend
- **Frankincense:** 3 drops
- **Sandalwood:** 1 to 3 drops
- **Carrot seed:** 1 drop

Frankincense oil is used in many skin-care formulas, as it helps to generate healthy tissue.

Diffuse

- *Shower:* This will help move the blood. Add a drop of the blend to a damp washcloth and fold the cloth so that the oils will not directly touch your skin. Gently press the cloth to the liver spots for a few minutes while you shower. Follow with a cool water splash or spritz.

- *Nebulizing diffuser:* If there are heat signs, such as redness or spider veins (see below), accompanying your liver spots, try holding the affected area over a nebulizing diffuser for several minutes several times a day. Follow with the topical treatment described below.

Topical Treatment

The Liver Spots blend also works well as a spot application in a base of rosehip oil. Use a ratio of 1 drop to ¼ teaspoon (1 mL) base oil.

Spider Veins

Spider veins, or telangiectasias, are little red bursts of enlarged or broken capillaries near the skin's surface that disappear momentarily when pressed and reappear when the blood rushes back. This blend may help the body reabsorb these nonfunctional veins.

Steam can irritate spider veins, so avoid using this blend in a facial steamer or shower.

Blend

- **Rose geranium:** 3 to 5 drops
- **Frankincense:** 3 drops
- **Helichrysum:** 1 drop

Diffuse

- *Ultrasonic diffuser:* Direct the mist toward your face or other affected body parts for several minutes several times a day.

Topical Treatment

Add the Spider Veins blend to sea buckthorn oil or rosehip oil for spot applications. Use a ratio of 1 drop blend to 10 drops base oil.

Dry Patches

Occasional dry patches that appear on the face, especially on combination skin, may benefit from this blend, which helps increase circulation and encourages moisture.

Blend
- **Frankincense:** 3 to 5 drops
- **Carrot seed:** 1 to 3 drops
- **Patchouli:** 1 drop

Diffuse

- *Ultrasonic or nebulizing diffuser:* Direct the mist toward the area of your face where the dry patches occur.

- *Facial steamer:* Set the steamer to its coolest setting, as heat generally exacerbates dryness. Add 1 to 3 drops of the blend to the steamer, depending on its size (follow the directions that accompany your steamer).

> ## Topical Treatment
>
> If you want to use the Dry Patches blend as a spot application, add it to macadamia nut oil at a ratio of 1 drop blend to 10 drops base oil.

A diffuser that creates a fine mist, such as an ultrasonic or nebulizing diffuser, works best for dry skin, but a warm steam is often well tolerated.

Red Irritated Patches

For red irritated patches anywhere on your skin, consider this cooling and soothing blend.

Blend
- **Lavender:** 3 to 5 drops
- **Blue chamomile:** 3 drops
- **Rose:** 1 drop

Diffuse
- *Ultrasonic diffuser:* Direct the mist toward the area of your skin where the red patches appear. Follow with the topical treatment suggested below.

Blue chamomile oil is cooling for inflammations of all kinds. Consider blue chamomile for any irritation of the skin.

> ## Topical Treatment
>
> Add the Red Irritated Patches blend to sea buckthorn oil to use as a spot application. Use a ratio of 1 to 3 drops blend to ¼ teaspoon (1 mL) base oil. Sea buckthorn is fantastic for reducing heat.

Postmenopausal Breakouts

Hormonal imbalances can cause skin breakouts at any time of life, including after menopause.

Blend
- **Sandalwood:** 1 to 3 drops
- **Clary sage:** 1 drop
- **Rose geranium:** 1 drop

Diffuse
- *Facial steamer:* Add 1 to 3 drops of the blend to the steamer, depending on its size (follow the directions that accompany your steamer).
- *Shower:* Add a few drops of the blend to a damp washcloth and fold the cloth so that the oils will not directly touch your skin. Gently press the cloth to the areas of breakout while you shower.

Clary sage is both cooling and moistening, making it a perfect oil for hot, dry conditions. It has a marked effect on hormonal imbalances.

Topical Treatment

Add 1 drop of the Postmenopausal Breakouts blend to 10 drops of jojoba oil and apply directly to the breakouts — preferably at night, as skin is in repair mode while we sleep.

Sagging Tissue

As we age, tissue loses it resiliency and becomes less toned. This blend can help!

Blend
- **Carrot seed:** 3 drops
- **Rose geranium:** 3 drops
- **Helichrysum:** 1 to 3 drops

Diffuse
- *Facial steamer:* Add 1 to 3 drops of the blend to the steamer, depending on its size (follow the directions that accompany your steamer).
- *Ultrasonic* or *nebulizing diffuser:* Direct the mist toward your area of concern for a few minutes a few times a day.

Tissue often sags because it is dehydrated, and warm steam can help with this.

For more information on these and other base oils, see Appendix 1 (page 198).

Top Base Oils for Aging Skin

- **Argan oil:** This rich, nurturing oil, also called Morocco oil, can significantly improve the tone of aging skin.
- **Avocado oil:** Although it is a very rich oil, avocado oil absorbs well into the skin. Consider adding a few drops of an essential oil blend to mashed avocado and using it as a mask. Be sure to mash well and blend thoroughly.
- **Macadamia nut oil:** This nut oil may strengthen thin tissue. It is well absorbed and does not leave a greasy residue.
- **Rosehip oil:** Rich in vitamin C, known to encourage healing of the skin, rosehip oil is truly miraculous for reducing the appearance of scars, wrinkles and discolorations.
- **Sea buckthorn oil:** Pressed from a brilliant orange fruit, this oil is especially wonderful for sunburn or any skin condition where there is heat.

Dry Skin

Dry skin can happen at any time of life, but definitely becomes more likely as we age! However, if we care for ourselves holistically, it is much less apt to become a problem.

It is worth noting that dull, dry skin may be an early warning sign of an internal imbalance. Other causes of dry skin include low water intake, poor-quality oils in the diet, chronic illness and emotional distress — shock, in particular, can very rapidly affect the skin in a noticeable way.

Single Oils

- Blue chamomile
- Carrot seed
- Frankincense
- Helichrysum
- Lavender
- Myrrh
- Patchouli
- Rose
- Rose geranium
- Sage
- Sandalwood

Deep and Dry Wrinkles

While many essential oil blends will help alleviate tiny lines, it is more difficult to address deep wrinkles that are well established. In effect, wrinkled tissue acts like scar tissue, unable to regenerate because of damage or overuse. This blend may help.

Blend
- **Helichrysum:** 3 drops
- **Patchouli:** 1 to 3 drops
- **Sage:** 1 drop

Diffuse
- *Facial steamer:* Add 1 to 3 drops of the blend to the steamer, depending on its size (follow the directions that accompany your steamer). Use daily for a maximum of 2 weeks, then switch to a more nourishing oil blend, like the Dry Mature Skin blend, page 156.

Patchouli has been used for a very long time in skin-care formulas, as it is amazingly effective at balancing dry, tired skin.

Topical Treatment

Add 1 drop of the Deep and Dry Wrinkles blend to ¼ teaspoon (1 mL) of rosehip oil and apply directly to the deep wrinkles. Be sure to use for only 2 weeks before switching to a more nourishing oil blend.

Dull Skin

Skin typically has a lovely luster, a sign of vitality we call an "inner glow." If your skin is looking dull, address the issue with changes to your diet and water intake, and this blend.

Blend
- **Helichrysum:** 3 drops
- **Carrot seed:** 1 drop
- **Patchouli:** 1 drop

Diffuse
- *Facial steamer:* Add 1 to 3 drops of the blend to the steamer, depending on its size (follow the directions that accompany your steamer).
- *Shower:* Add 1 drop of the blend to a damp washcloth and fold the cloth so that the oils will not directly touch your skin. Place the cloth over your face for a moment or two while you shower.

> When using a facial steamer, remember that it is very important to keep your eyes closed throughout.

Dry Mature Skin

Although it's often due to a lack of care over time, dryness in mature skin can also be hormonally induced (see also Menopause, page 108). Don't despair! Noticeable results can be achieved with regular applications of this blend.

Blend
- **Frankincense:** 3 drops
- **Rose or rose geranium:** 1 drop
- **Sandalwood:** 1 drop

Diffuse
- *Facial steamer:* Add 1 to 3 drops of the blend to the steamer, depending on its size (follow the directions that accompany your steamer).

> The Dry Mature Skin blend is an incredibly effective moisturizer and smells divine!

Topical Treatment

If your dry skin is due to changes in hormonal status, add the Dry Mature Skin blend to evening primrose oil or macadamia nut oil — 1 to 3 drops blend to 1 teaspoon (5 mL) base oil — and apply as a topical treatment.

Eczema

Eczema is always a sign of a greater underlying imbalance that needs to be addressed before the skin condition will resolve. In the meantime, this blend may help alleviate the irritation and itch.

Blend
- **Lavender:** 3 to 5 drops
- **Blue chamomile:** 3 drops
- **Myrrh:** 1 drop

Diffuse
- *Shower:* Add 1 to 3 drops of the blend to a damp washcloth and fold the cloth so that the oils will not directly touch your skin. Gently press the cloth to the affected skin while you shower.

Topical Treatment

The Eczema blend also works well as a spot application. Add 1 to 3 drops of the blend to 1 teaspoon (5 mL) of almond or avocado oil.

Avocado oil is deeply nourishing to the skin, and is one of the few fruit sources of fat. A topical application of mashed avocado works well for treating eczema!

Oily Skin

Skin often becomes oily during times of hormonal changes, such as puberty or menopause, and oil production may also increase during a woman's monthly menstrual cycle. Try using these essential oils to help balance excessively oily skin.

Single Oils

- Basil
- Clary sage
- Eucalyptus citriodora
- Lavender
- Lemon
- Peppermint
- Rose
- Rose geranium

Contrary to common belief, oily food does not make the skin oily (although it can lead to other problems), especially if the food is prepared using healthful oils like olive or sunflower oil.

Hormonal Flux

The essential oils in this blend have a history of successfully balancing hormones during hormonal shifts.

Blend
- **Lavender:** 3 to 5 drops
- **Clary sage:** 3 drops
- **Rose geranium:** 3 drops

Diffuse
- *Facial steamer:* Add 1 to 3 drops of the blend to the steamer, depending on its size (follow the directions that accompany your steamer).
- *Shower:* Add a drop of the blend to a damp washcloth and fold the cloth so that the oils do not directly touch your skin. Gently press the cloth to your face for a few minutes while you shower.

Topical Treatment

To use the Hormonal Flux blend as a spot treatment, add 1 drop to ¼ teaspoon (1 mL) of base oil, such as hazelnut oil, and apply to oily patches.

Balancing Abuse

Sometimes we unintentionally abuse our skin by using the wrong products (see Skip the Strippers, page 159). After you stop using whatever products may have led to increased oil production, try this blend to bring your skin back into balance.

Rose oil's moisturizing properties make it very useful in skin-care blends.

Blend
- **Lavender:** 3 to 5 drops
- **Eucalyptus citriodora:** 3 drops
- **Rose:** 1 drop

Diffuse

- *Facial steamer:* Add 1 to 3 drops of the blend to the steamer, depending on its size (follow the directions that accompany your steamer).

- *Shower:* Add a drop of the blend to a damp washcloth and fold the cloth so that the oils do not directly touch your skin. Gently press the cloth to your face for a few minutes while you shower.

Topical Treatment

Create a serum by adding a drop or two of the Balancing Abuse blend to ¼ teaspoon (1 mL) of a mild base oil, such as jojoba oil. Apply a thin layer over oily areas.

Refresh!

Sometimes it just feels good to remove the excess oil from your skin. This blend will remove oil without stripping, but be sure to immediately follow up with a balancing oil blend, like the Hormonal Flux blend (page 158).

Blend

- **Basil:** 1 to 3 drops
- **Lemon:** 1 drop
- **Peppermint:** 1 drop

Diffuse

- *Facial steamer:* Add 1 to 3 drops of the blend to the steamer, depending on its size (follow the directions that accompany your steamer).

- *Shower:* Add a few drops of the blend to a damp washcloth and fold the cloth so that the oils will not directly touch your skin. Gently press the cloth to the oily areas while you shower.

When using a facial steamer, remember that it is very important to keep your eyes closed throughout.

Skip the Strippers

Do not use soap-based cleansers! They are usually stripping. When the skin is stripped of its natural oils, oil production goes into overdrive and compounds the problem. Interestingly, an oil-based cleanser is best. Many people with oily skin find coconut oil to be very effective; try adding a bit of French green clay, which is absorptive without being stripping.

Rashes

The skin is an emunctory organ, meaning it is capable of clearing toxins from the body. A rash is often a sign of an underlying issue within the body, as the body attempts to resolve the issue by taking advantage of the skin's toxin-clearing ability. Topical steroids usually make things worse, as they prevent the skin's natural clearing action by suppressing the symptoms. Essential oils, on the other hand, encourage the clearing function, helping the body heal while also relieving the irritating symptoms.

Single Oils

- Basil
- Blue chamomile
- Clove
- Eucalyptus citriodora
- Lavender
- Patchouli
- Peppermint
- Ravintsara
- Rose geranium
- Sandalwood
- Tea tree

Blue chamomile oil is cooling for inflammations of all kinds. Consider blue chamomile for any irritation of the skin.

Allergic Rash

Many allergy attacks are accompanied by an itchy rash. This blend can help stop the itch and soothe the skin.

Blend

- **Lavender:** 3 to 5 drops
- **Eucalyptus citriodora:** 1 to 3 drops
- **Blue chamomile:** 1 drop

Diffuse

- *Nebulizing or ultrasonic diffuser:* For a rash associated with a lot of heat signs, like redness and/or cracked skin, direct the mist toward the area where the rash occurs.

- *Inhalation stick:* Use as needed. Inhaling the oils may help reduce the reactivity of the system as a whole by calming an overactive immune response.

- *Shower:* Apply a few drops of the blend to a damp washcloth and fold the cloth so that the oils will not directly touch your skin. Gently press the cloth to the affected areas while you shower.

Hives

Try this blend to help soothe allergic urticaria, also known as hives.

Be sure to use sandalwood oil that comes from an ethically harvested source.

Blend

- **Lavender:** 5 to 8 drops
- **Sandalwood:** 1 to 3 drops
- **Basil:** 1 drop

Diffuse

- *Shower:* Add a few drops of the blend to a warm, wet washcloth and take it into the shower with you. Allow the oils to diffuse into the steam of the shower for a while, then moisten the cloth and fold it so that the oils will not directly touch your skin. Gently rub the cloth over areas of itchy skin.

Topical Treatment

The Hives blend can also be added to jojoba oil and applied directly to the skin. Use a ratio of 5 drops blend per ¼ teaspoon (1 mL) jojoba oil.

Plant-Induced Rash

If you come into contact with a plant whose oils cause a rash, such as poison ivy, oak or sumac, the most important response is to remove all traces of the oil (actually a resin called urushiol) from your skin as soon as possible. A combination of soap and warm water works well. Rubbing alcohol may also help if you are unable to use soap and water.

Once you are sure all of the urushiol has been removed, try this essential oil blend to reduce the likelihood of blistering and itchiness.

Blend

- **Lavender:** 3 to 5 drops
- **Basil:** 1 to 3 drops
- **Peppermint:** 1 drop

Never treat a plant-induced rash before removing urushiol from your skin, or the treatment may actually end up making things worse.

Diffuse

- *Shower:* Apply 1 to 3 drops of the blend to a damp washcloth and fold the cloth so that the oils will not directly touch your skin. Gently press the cloth to all areas of affected skin while you shower.

Bug Bites

Stop the itch quickly with this simple topical blend:

- Blue chamomile: 3 drops
- Lavender: 3 drops
- Tea tree: 1 drop

This one really needs to be applied to the skin to be effective. It is probably the only oil blend I would ever consider applying undiluted to the skin, as it is quite safe and is more effective that way. Place a drop of the blend on a cotton bud and dab onto the bites as needed.

Shingles

Shingles is an imbalance caused by a virus that lives in the nerve root. When the virus becomes activated, it can cause extreme pain and sensitivity wherever those nerves run. This blend will help decrease nerve sensitivity and reduce the viral load.

Blend

- **Eucalyptus citriodora:** 3 to 5 drops
- **Ravintsara:** 3 drops
- **Rose geranium:** 3 drops

In place of the eucalyptus oil, you can use 1 drop of clove oil in the Shingles blend.

Diffuse

- *Nebulizing diffuser:* The increased exposure to the essential oil molecules provided by the nebulized mist is helpful here. Direct the mist toward the affected area.

- *Shower:* Apply up to 5 drops of the blend to a damp washcloth and fold the cloth so that the oils will not directly touch your skin. Gently press the cloth to the blistered areas of skin while you shower.

Topical Treatment

Add up to 5 drops of the Shingles blend to ¼ teaspoon (1 mL) of a base oil — coconut oil is a good choice here, as it has been shown to have antiviral properties.

Headaches

Headaches occur for many different reasons and can affect many different parts of the head and even the neck. For example, cluster headaches often appear around one eye, while a vertex headache usually feels like a stabbing point of pain at the very top of the head. Because each type of headache has a different etiology, or root cause, each will benefit from different essential oils and blends.

All headache types benefit from hydration and relaxation, so when a headache strikes, try to drink water and sit quietly in a darkened room. Foot baths are also helpful for nearly all headaches, although perhaps less so with migraines. Most of these blends can be added directly to a foot bath, a few drops at a time, to help reduce the pain and pressure of a headache.

Single Oils

- Black pepper
- Blue chamomile
- Clary sage
- Eucalyptus globulus
- Ginger
- Helichrysum
- Lavender
- Melissa
- Peppermint
- Rose geranium
- Rosemary
- Sage
- Spikenard
- Vetiver

Foot Baths and Headaches

With most headaches, the issue is congested blood in the head. Helping the blood move out of the head and into the other extremities can help reduce the pain. Using a warming substance, such as mustard powder, in a foot bath — 1 tablespoon (15 mL) to a full bath — will dilate the blood vessels of the lower limbs, allowing for increased flow in that direction. Placing a peppermint oil compress on the back of the neck will constrict the blood vessels to the head, helping to move the stagnant blood out of the head and into the rest of the body. This combination can work wonders! Avoid this treatment if you tend to have low blood pressure.

Migraine

Despite years of research, migraines are still something of a mystery. Recent studies show that the amount of certain amino acids in the body increases during a migraine, offering a new direction toward finding a cure. Until this disease (or cluster of symptoms, really) is understood, the oils below can help ward off a potential migraine and reduce the severity once it hits.

The Migraine blend may be effective for all types of headaches.

A Word of Caution

In rare cases, migraine sufferers report that scents trigger or worsen a migraine, although this is usually due to synthetic fragrances. Still, be cautious when first using essential oils to treat a migraine!

Blend
- **Lavender:** 8 to 10 drops
- **Blue chamomile:** 1 drop
- **Peppermint:** 1 drop

Diffuse
- *Nebulizing diffuser:* Use in a dark, quiet room at the first hint of prodromal (precursor) symptoms.
- *Inhalation stick:* Because migraines can strike anytime, it is a good idea to carry one of these at all times to use as needed.

Topical Treatment

At the first sign of prodromal symptoms, such as fatigue, irritability or visual auras, add 3 drops of the Migraine blend to ½ teaspoon (2 mL) hempseed oil and massage into the neck and head.

Tension Headache

Tension headaches are probably more common than any other type. As the name indicates, the pain is caused by tension, usually in the neck and shoulders. Many sufferers describe a tension headache as feeling like a tight band around the head.

Be aware that both ginger and black pepper can cause or increase redness as the oils work to move the blood.

Blend
- **Ginger:** 3 to 5 drops
- **Black pepper:** 1 drop
- **Helichrysum:** 1 drop

Diffuse

- *Nebulizing diffuser:* Diffuse for a few minutes at the first sign of tension.

- *Shower:* Add a few drops of the blend to a damp washcloth and fold the cloth so that the oils will not directly touch your skin. As you shower, alternate gently pressing the cloth to the back of your neck and to your forehead.

Topical Treatment

Add 1 drop of the Tension Headache blend to ¼ teaspoon (1 mL) base oil, such as sunflower oil, and massage into the head and neck.

Sinus Headache

Because this type of headache is often the result of a sinus infection, the oils recommended here both open and clear infectious agents from the sinuses. This blend is effective for the pain of sinus congestion from allergies or a cold as well.

Blend

- **Eucalyptus globulus:** 3 drops
- **Helichrysum:** 1 to 3 drops
- **Peppermint:** 1 drop

Diffuse

- *Ultrasonic diffuser:* Diffuse for a few minutes several times a day, especially if infection or heat signs, like redness, accompany your sinus headache. The cool mist ensures you are not compounding the problem by adding heat.

- *Shower:* Add a few drops of the blend to a damp washcloth and fold the cloth so that the oils will not directly touch your skin. As you shower, alternate gently pressing the cloth to your frontal sinuses and to your forehead.

- *Inhalation stick:* Use as needed, and use often during the acute phase of congestion.

Some holistic practitioners add a drop of the Sinus Headache blend to a cotton bud and insert it into the nostril. If you decide to try this, be very careful! These are strong oils and can cause a strong reaction. Also, be sure not to insert the bud too far into the nose — most practitioners use extra-long swabs that can get far into the cavity without getting stuck, but it is quite easy to lose your grasp on a small cotton bud.

Hormonal Headache

This blend is especially effective if your headaches are a common symptom of monthly hormonal shifts. It may also be helpful for headaches that occur during perimenopause and postmenopause.

If your headaches follow a predictable pattern around the time of your period, try to use this blend *before* the day the headaches typically first occur (often a day or two before the onset of menses).

Blend
- **Melissa or lavender:** 3 to 5 drops
- **Clary sage:** 1 to 3 drops
- **Rose geranium:** 1 to 3 drops

Diffuse
- *Nebulizing diffuser:* Turn it on when you go to bed and set a timer to ensure that it runs for only about 15 minutes.

- *Personal diffuser,* such as an inhalation stick. Use frequently at the first sign of a headache, but do not use for more than a day or two at a time.

Topical Treatment

This blend can also be added to a base of evening primrose oil, using a ratio of 1 drop blend to ¼ teaspoon (1 mL) base oil. Apply to the temples, the forehead or the back of the neck — wherever the pain typically occurs.

Cluster Headaches

These headaches usually appear in a succession, with each episode lasting around 15 minutes, although some people experience pain for several hours. They may strike for several days or months, with long periods of no headaches at all.

Cluster headaches are often one-sided and may be accompanied by other symptoms, like redness or eye pain.

Blend
- **Rosemary:** 1 to 3 drops
- **Sage:** 1 drop
- **Spikenard:** 1 drop

Diffuse
- *Fan diffuser* or *nebulizing diffuser:* If the spikenard oil is viscous (which depends on the harvest), use a fan diffuser; if it is thin, a nebulizing diffuser is best. Diffuse for a few minutes at the first sign of pain.

- *Personal diffuser:* Smelling salts are a good option here. Carry the blend at all times — because the cluster moves through in waves, the occurrences may be a little unpredictable, so it's best to be prepared.

- *Shower:* Add a few drops of the blend to a damp washcloth and fold the cloth so that the oils will not directly touch your skin. Gently press the cloth to the back of your neck while you shower.

Vertex Headache

These headaches occur at the very top of the head, called the vertex, and often feel sharp and stabbing. The oils in this blend help move the blood out of the head, and are especially effective if added to a foot bath.

Blend
- **Helichrysum:** 1 to 3 drops
- **Vetiver:** 1 to 3 drops
- **Spikenard:** 1 drop

Diffuse
- *Foot bath:* Add a few drops of the blend to a warm foot bath. Relax with your feet in the bath and a cloth over your eyes to block out the light.

- *Nebulizing diffuser:* Diffuse for a few minutes at the first sign of pain.

While enjoying your foot bath, you can use a peppermint oil compress on the back of your neck as well, but be sure to fold the compress in such a way that the oil does not directly touch your skin.

Topical Treatment

If you do not have time for a foot bath, add the Vertex Headache blend to a base of sunflower oil and apply to your feet. Use a ratio of 1 to 3 drops blend to $\frac{1}{4}$ teaspoon (1 mL) base oil. Keep a small vial of this mixture to apply as needed. You can also use it on your ankles if you cannot apply it to your feet.

Hemorrhoids

There is no discomfort quite like that of hemorrhoids. Everything is uncomfortable: sitting, lying down — even standing does not relieve the pain.

Hemorrhoids, a condition of weakened veins, are classified as internal (in the lower rectum) or external (around the anus). It is quite easy to address the discomfort of external hemorrhoids by diffusing essential oils, and it is worth taking the time to do so, as the pain and swelling can be significantly reduced.

This is a condition that definitely benefits from lifestyle changes! In particular, choose foods that encourage easy evacuation and increase exercise. Exercise is important because veins require the actions of the surrounding muscles to pump blood back up to the heart.

A word about rectal prolapse: while this is not the same as hemorrhoids, it is often mistaken for that condition. Be sure to have a doctor confirm that the issue is hemorrhoids before addressing the symptoms.

Heavy Bleeding

If there is a lot of bleeding from the hemorrhoids, this blend will help. The oils are primarily astringing, and encourage healing at the site.

Blend
- **Cypress:** 3 to 5 drops
- **Frankincense:** 3 to 5 drops
- **Bay laurel:** 1 to 3 drops

Diffuse

- *Steaming chair:* This is an excellent way to deliver the benefits of essential oils directly to the affected area. Add 3 to 5 drops of the blend to the water in the steaming bowl and sit over it for at least 15 minutes. This can be repeated up to three times a day for up to a month. If no benefits are seen, discontinue use.

- *Sitz bath:* Use as much water as possible, remembering that much of it will be displaced when you sit down. Add 3 to 5 drops of the blend before sitting in the bath.

Be aware that if there is heavy bleeding, the blood will stain the water. On the other hand, the oils in the Heavy Bleeding blend are known to help stop bleeding. If the bleeding does not slow or stop within 30 minutes, visit your doctor.

Itching

Having an itchy bum is bad enough, but with hemorrhoids, scratching is out of the question. Soothe the itch with this blend.

Blend

- **Lavender:** 3 to 5 drops
- **German or blue chamomile:** 1 drop
- **Rose geranium:** 1 drop

Diffuse

- *Steaming chair:* Add 3 to 5 drops of the blend to the water in the steaming bowl and sit over it for at least 15 minutes. This can be repeated up to three times a day for up to a month. If no benefits are seen, discontinue use.

- *Spritzer:* Add the entire blend to a base of 2 tablespoons (30 mL) of aloe vera juice or extremely diluted apple cider vinegar or witch hazel — 1 tablespoon (15 mL) in ½ to 1 cup (125 to 250 mL) of water. Shake well, then spritz the affected area as needed.

Be sure to patch-test your spritz first if you choose to use aloe vera juice — some people are sensitive to aloe and find it drying.

Protective Barrier

This blend may be the only one that is not wonderful in a steam diffusion, as the oils are dense and less likely to diffuse into steam. Instead, make it into a topical treatment, using coconut or jojoba oil as a base, to form a barrier between the irritated tissue and the irritation of clothing:

- Frankincense: 3 drops
- Myrrh: 1 drop
- Peru balsam: 1 drop

Add the oils to ¼ to ½ tsp (1 to 2 mL) of the base oil. Be sure to apply at least 30 minutes before dressing, to avoid staining.

Scar Tissue

It is very difficult for the perianal skin to heal in the presence of ongoing inflammation; scar tissue often forms instead. This blend may help soften scarring and encourage new healthy tissue.

Blend
- **Helichrysum:** 3 drops
- **Sandalwood:** 3 drops
- **Sage:** 1 drop

Diffuse

- *Steaming chair:* Add 3 to 5 drops of the blend to the water in the steaming bowl and sit over it for at least 15 minutes. This can be repeated up to three times a day for up to a month. If no benefits are seen, discontinue use.

- *Sitz bath:* Use as much water as possible, remembering that much of it will be displaced when you sit down. Add 1 to 3 drops of the blend before sitting in the bath.

When you're preparing a sitz bath, adding 1 to 3 drops of the blend to an emulsifying agent, such as a pinch of lecithin, can help to incorporate the oils into the water.

Stagnant Blood

In Chinese medicine, hemorrhoids may be seen as a condition called "stagnant blood." If there are more blue or purple veins and less bleeding, this blend may be the best choice, as the oils are known to help encourage circulation. The peppermint helps cool the heat, too.

Blend
- **Carrot seed:** 3 drops
- **Helichrysum:** 3 drops
- **Peppermint:** 1 drop

Diffuse

- *Steaming chair:* Add 3 to 5 drops of the blend to the water in the steaming bowl and sit over it for at least 15 minutes. This can be repeated up to three times a day for up to a month. If no benefits are seen, discontinue use.

- *Spritzer:* Add the entire blend to a base of 2 tablespoons (30 mL) of aloe vera juice or extremely diluted apple cider vinegar or witch hazel — 1 tablespoon (15 mL) in ½ to 1 cup (125 to 250 mL) of water. Shake well, then spritz the affected area as needed.

You can store the spritzer in the fridge for even more cooling power. Keep in mind that spritzer blends are best used up in a week or less, so make small amounts.

Infected Tissue

For obvious reasons, it is quite easy for a hemorrhoid to become infected. The oils in this blend are strongly antimicrobial and encourage blood and accompanying immune factors to move into the area.

Blend

- **Lavender:** 5 drops
- **Helichrysum:** 1 drop
- **Thyme:** 1 drop

Diffuse

- *Steaming chair:* Add 3 to 5 drops of the blend to the water in the steaming bowl and sit over it for at least 15 minutes. This can be repeated up to three times a day for up to a month. If no benefits are seen, discontinue use.

- *Spritzer:* Add the entire blend to a base of 2 tablespoons (30 mL) of aloe vera juice or extremely diluted apple cider vinegar or witch hazel — 1 tablespoon (15 mL) in $\frac{1}{2}$ to 1 cup (125 to 250 mL) of water. Shake well, then spritz the affected area as needed.

Topical Treatment

Cotton facial pads, often recommended in this book for passive diffusion (see page 21), can also be used for topical applications. Add a drop or two of the Stagnant Blood blend or the Infected Tissue blend to aloe vera juice or cooled herbal tea, such as chamomile or peppermint. (Peppermint tea can also be used in this way on its own.) Soak a cotton pad in the mixture and apply topically.

Soothe the Pain

This blend can be used alone or added to any of the others to address the pain. Be sure to compensate for the additional oils and cut back on the amount of each blend used when diffusing.

Blend

- **Lavender:** 8 to 10 drops
- **Rose geranium:** 3 to 5 drops
- **Bay laurel:** 1 drop

Diffuse

- *Steaming chair:* Add 3 to 5 drops of the blend to the water in the steaming bowl and sit over it for at least 15 minutes. This can be repeated up to three times a day for up to a month. If no benefits are seen, discontinue use.

Pain is almost always accompanied by inflammation, especially at first. Bay laurel is an astringing essential oil that helps tone the boggy tissue associated with inflammation.

Topical Treatment

Add the Soothe the Pain blend to a base oil at a ratio of 3 drops blend to $\frac{1}{2}$ teaspoon (2 mL) base oil. Consider using tamanu oil as the base, as it is spectacularly effective at reducing pain.

Infectious Diseases

Single Oils

- Anise
- Bay laurel
- Carrot seed
- Cinnamon
- Clary sage
- Clove
- Eucalyptus citriodora
- Eucalyptus globulus
- Eucalyptus radiata
- Frankincense
- Ginger
- Grapefruit
- Lavender
- Lemon
- Lemongrass
- Melissa
- Myrrh
- Oregano
- Patchouli
- Peppermint
- Ravintsara
- Rose geranium
- Rosemary
- Sweet orange
- Thyme
- Thyme linalool

This is a very large and broad category, but most infectious diseases can be treated similarly, as so many essential oils are multifunctional — the same oils that work to reduce viral loads are often helpful against fungus, for example.

Infections can be viral, bacterial or fungal. Generally speaking, milder, more common conditions, like a cold or a stomach bug, are viral. Bacterial infections, such as gangrene or botulism, tend to be much more serious, and may even be life-threatening. Fungal infections are mainly irritating and persistent. There are more-threatening fungal infections, but they are usually found only in patients with a severely compromised immune system.

Viral Infections

See also the Shingles blend (page 162).

Clean Surfaces!

Viruses can live on surfaces for quite a long time. Adding essential oils to very diluted vinegar and using it to clean surfaces is a remarkably effective way to kill many viruses. The citrus oils, in particular, have a great reputation for this use.

Reproductive Infections

Viral infections of the reproductive system are usually either herpes or vaginitis. Melissa (lemon balm) has an incredible track record for effectively treating herpes. Thyme and oregano are also very effective, but must be used in tiny amounts.

Blend
- **Rose geranium:** 5 to 8 drops
- **Melissa:** 1 drop
- **Thyme:** 1 drop

Diffuse

- *Steaming chair:* This is an excellent way to deliver the benefits of essential oils directly to the affected area. Add 3 to 5 drops of the blend to the water in the steaming bowl and sit over it for at least 15 minutes. This can be repeated up to three times a day for up to a month. If no benefits are seen, discontinue use.

- *Sitz bath:* Use as much water as possible, remembering that much of it will be displaced when you sit down. Add 1 to 3 drops of the blend before sitting in the bath. Use as needed, at least once a day.

- *Spritzer:* Add the entire blend to ¼ cup (60 mL) of distilled water. Shake well, then spritz the affected area as needed.

Gastrointestinal Virus

This is the condition commonly called "stomach flu," even though it is not the influenza virus that causes the problem! The oils in this blend will go a long way toward settling the stomach, whether the culprit is a viral infection or food poisoning.

The Gastrointestinal Virus blend is also incredibly effective in capsule form, and encapsulated versions of all three oils are readily available in health food stores.

Blend

- **Ginger:** 1 drop
- **Oregano:** 1 drop
- **Peppermint:** 1 drop

Diffuse

- *Nebulizing diffuser, ultrasonic diffuser or humidifier:* Run several times a day for a few minutes at a time.

Healing Help

A ginger or peppermint tea can also help. If nothing is staying down, consider turning the tea into ice, as ice chips are often well tolerated.

Liver Infections

If you have a viral infection of the liver, such as hepatitis, diffusing this blend in your living space on a regular basis may help.

Blend
- **Eucalyptus citriodora:** 5 drops
- **Rosemary:** 3 drops
- **Carrot seed:** 1 drop

Diffuse
- *Nebulizing diffuser, ultrasonic diffuser or humidifier:* Run several times a day for a few minutes at a time.
- *Shower:* Add 1 drop to a damp washcloth and fold the cloth so the oils will not touch your skin. Press gently over the liver (under the ribs on the right side of your body).

> ### Topical Treatment
> The Liver Infections blend is most effective if added to a base oil, such as hazelnut or olive oil, and massaged directly over the liver. Use a ratio of 5 drops blend to 1 teaspoon (5 mL) base oil.

Carrot seed oil has a particular affinity for the liver, and can help clear toxins.

Respiratory Infections

This blend can help ease breathing, soothe a raw throat and reduce the cough reflex. For the eucalyptus, use eucalyptus globulus when treating adults and eucalyptus radiata for kids. (See also "Respiratory Health," pages 126–145.)

Blend
- **Eucalyptus globulus or radiata:** 8 to 10 drops
- **Ravintsara:** 3 drops
- **Clove or bay laurel:** 1 drop

Diffuse
- *Nebulizing diffuser* in the sick room for 5 to 10 minutes at a time.
- *Facial steamer:* This method will effectively deliver the blend exactly where it needs to go. Add 1 to 3 drops of the blend, depending on the size of your steamer's well.
- *Personal nebulizing diffuser:* Use with great care, as the oils in this blend are very strong. Introduce it slowly, especially if breathing is already difficult.

Clove oil is more effective than bay laurel oil for respiratory infections, and is safe for children, but some people find it overwhelming.

Common Cold

You can rely on eucalyptus. Specifically, eucalyptus globulus for adults and eucalyptus radiata for kids. Both are strongly antiviral, but eucalyptus radiata is milder. The oils in the blends below are all very effective against bacteria and fungi, too.

Blend for Adults
- **Eucalyptus globulus:** 3 drops
- **Cinnamon:** 1 drop
- **Peppermint:** 1 drop

Blend for Children
- **Sweet orange:** 3 drops
- **Eucalyptus radiata:** 1 drop
- **Thyme linalool:** 1 drop

The Sinus Headache blend (page 165) may be helpful for clearing out the clogged sinuses that often accompany a cold.

Diffuse
- *Nebulizing diffuser* in the sick room for 5 to 10 minutes at a time.

- *Humidifiers* also do a great job here, as warm, moist air generally helps a cold sufferer.

- *Facial steamer:* This method will effectively deliver the blend exactly where it needs to go. Add 1 to 3 drops of the blend, depending on the size of your steamer's well.

Bacterial Infections

For more severe bacterial infections, see a doctor as soon as possible. Timely treatment is often the key to successful treatment.

Minor bacterial infections on the surface of the body are quite easily treated with essential oils and acupressure. Almost all essential oils are antibacterial, although some are extremely potent and can damage tissue if not used carefully. One drop of essential oil diluted in 1 teaspoon (5 mL) of base oil (1% dilution) is effective and safe, but definitely do a patch-test first (see page 77).

When there is a larger area of tissue affected (for example, a large abrasion that has become infected), another option is to use fresh thyme and/or oregano to make a wash: in a small bowl, steep a small handful of herbs in 1 cup (250 mL) of water. The steeped herbs can also be wrapped in muslin and applied directly to the wound as an herb pack.

MRSA

A frightening bacterial infection — MRSA (methicillin-resistant *Staphylococcus aureus*) — is on the rise. Fortunately, essential oils show great promise for treating it. Lemongrass, neroli, clove and thuja, in particular, seem to be very effective against staph aureus overgrowth.

Fungal Infections

Some of the more common fungal infections are candida, tinea and nail fungus.

Vaginal Candida

Candida most commonly occurs vaginally but can happen anywhere. The oils in this blend are known to be effective against candida.

Candida responds best to a change in diet. Avoid all sugar, yeast and mold-containing foods, like blue cheese, until symptoms abate. Be cautious when reintroducing these foods. Increasing fresh vegetables can help candida clear faster.

Blend
- **Lavender:** 8 to 10 drops
- **Rose geranium:** 5 drops
- **Clary sage:** 3 drops

Diffuse

- *Steaming chair:* This is an excellent way to deliver the benefits of essential oils directly to the affected area. Add 3 to 5 drops of the blend to the water in the steaming bowl and sit over it for at least 15 minutes. This can be repeated up to three times a day for up to a month. If no benefits are seen, discontinue use.

- *Sitz bath:* Use as much water as possible, remembering that much of it will be displaced when you sit down. Add 1 to 3 drops of the blend before sitting in the bath. Use as needed, at least once a day.

Thrush

This blend helps reduce the microbes that lead to thrush, a candida infection of the throat.

Blend

- **Myrrh:** 3 drops
- **Rose geranium:** 3 drops
- **Clove:** 1 drop

Diffuse

- *Facial steamer:* Breathe through a wide funnel or a paper cone to direct the steam specifically into the mouth, as these are quite harsh oils. Test carefully by allowing a tiny bit of the steam into your mouth before inhaling, to ensure you do not react negatively to it. Use several times a day.

- *Personal nebulizing diffuser:* Test carefully before inhaling, as described above. Use several times a day.

Healing Help

The Thrush blend can also be made into a mouthwash to be gargled several times a day. First, create a salt-water gargle by adding ¼ teaspoon (1 mL) of salt to 1 cup (250 mL) of warm water, stirring to dissolve the salt. Add no more than 4 drops of the oil blend to the salt-water base.

Be sure to keep your eyes closed when using a facial steamer.

Nipple Treatment

Thrush is very common in babies, as they will put anything in their mouths! And the fungus can be transferred to a mom's nipples during breastfeeding. If this happens, the nipples will need to be treated or the thrush will never resolve. You can make a topical treatment from the Thrush blend, but replace the clove oil with 1 to 3 drops of tea tree oil. Add the blend to a coconut oil base, using a ratio of 3 drops blend to ¼ teaspoon (1 mL) coconut oil, and apply regularly, at least 1 hour before and 30 minutes after breastfeeding.

Athlete's Foot

The Tinea pedis *fungus has a particular affinity for the feet. The blend below has a history of effectively preventing and combating it.*

Thyme is strongly medicinal in action. It can also be harsh and irritating, so it is best used in tiny amounts.

Blend

- **Rose geranium:** 5 drops
- **Peppermint:** 1 drop
- **Thyme:** 1 drop

Diffuse

- *Foot bath:* Add a few drops of the blend to a warm foot bath.
- *Spritzer:* Add the entire blend to 2 tablespoons (30 mL) of water in the spritzer bottle (or double both amounts). Shake well and spray on bath shoes, tennis shoes, shower floors — anywhere you might come in contact with the fungus.

Topical Treatment

As tinea often leads to dry, cracked skin, be sure to use a lubricating lotion or cream as well. You can try adding a drop of the Athlete's Foot blend to the lotion. Remember: less is more!

Jock Itch

Tinea cruris *is a fungus with an affinity for the groin. This blend can help wipe it out!*

Blend

- **Rose geranium:** 5 to 8 drops
- **Lemongrass:** 5 drops
- **Patchouli:** 1 drop

Diffuse

- *Steaming chair:* Add 3 to 5 drops of the blend to the water in the steaming bowl and sit over it for at least 15 minutes. This can be repeated up to three times a day for up to a month. If no benefits are seen, discontinue use.
- *Spritzer:* Add the entire blend to 2 tablespoons (30 mL) of water in the spritzer bottle (or double both amounts). Shake well and spray on the affected area as often as needed.

If you don't have a steaming chair, try sitting on a slatted stool over a steam bowl. These stools are commercially available for use in the bathroom or spa.

Topical Treatment

Adding the Jock Itch blend to 2 tablespoons (30 mL) of lotion and applying in small amounts directly to the rash can be very helpful.

Ringworm on the Head

Tinea capitis *is a fungus with an affinity for the scalp. This blend is very useful if applied regularly.*

Blend

- **Rose geranium:** 5 to 8 drops
- **Eucalyptus (any type):** 3 drops
- **Rosemary:** 1 to 3 drops

Diffuse

- *Shower:* Adding this blend to your shampoo can be very effective.

Topical Treatment

Add the Ringworm on the Head blend to 2 tablespoons (30 mL) of a base oil, such as jojoba oil, and apply directly to the scalp.

If you do not care for one of the oils used in a particular blend, simply omit it.

Ringworm of the Body

Tinea corporis *is a fungus that can colonize anywhere on the body. Try this blend for relief.*

Blend

- **Rose geranium:** 5 to 8 drops
- **Lemongrass:** 3 to 5 drops
- **Patchouli:** 1 to 3 drops

Diffuse

- *Nebulizing diffuser:* Run in the bathroom for the duration of your shower.
- *Shower:* Add a few drops of the blend to a damp washcloth and fold the cloth so that the oils will not directly touch your skin. Gently press the cloth to the affected areas while you shower.

Topical Treatment

Add the Ringworm of the Body blend to 2 tablespoons (30 mL) of lotion and apply small amounts to the affected areas.

Fungal infections are commonly transmitted at gyms and spas — places that are warm and moist, and where you might come in contact with people who carry the fungus. Take the appropriate precautions: wear bath shoes in the shower, use an antifungal soap (like tea tree) and dry yourself thoroughly. Applying cornstarch to areas that stay moist, like the underarms, may help.

Nail Fungus

Because of the anaerobic environment under the nails, on both the fingers and toes, fungi really thrive there. Nail fungus is notoriously hard to eradicate, but this blend is worth a try.

Blend
- **Eucalyptus globulus:** 5 to 8 drops
- **Cinnamon:** 1 drop
- **Thyme:** 1 drop

Diffuse

- *Nebulizing diffuser:* As a preventive measure, run the diffuser in the shower (or at the spa, if the owners are amenable to the idea) to stop the growth at the site of transference.

- *Spritzer:* Add the entire blend to 2 tablespoons (30 mL) of water in the spritzer bottle (or double both amounts). Shake well and spray on your bath shoes at the spa before wearing them, either as a preventive measure or as a treatment (and to help you avoid transferring the fungus to others).

- *Foot bath:* Add the entire blend to the bath and soak your nails several times a day for at least 30 minutes at a time.

Spritzes are best used up within a week or less, so make small amounts.

Topical Treatment

The Nail Fungus blend can also be applied directly to the nails, but use caution, as these oils are very caustic. Use a barrier cream around the cuticles to protect your skin.

Enhancing Your Environment with Essential Oils

Environmental Health Is Personal Health

The world around you … is you!

This chapter is devoted to scenting your environment rather than addressing personal health imbalances. In a very real way, though, it *is* about personal health, as our environment plays a huge — and often overlooked — role in our health on every level. If your surroundings are toxic because of mold issues, for example, your immune system is constantly being taxed, as it spends an enormous amount of time fighting the effects of the mold on your body.

But enhancing your environment also means improving your mental and emotional state. If you are constantly under stress at work, or are emotionally distressed at home, you are simply unable to be your healthiest, no matter how clean your surroundings may be. While no essential oil or blend can cure us of stress or make us happy, regular oil diffusion can absolutely lessen the effects of stress and distress on our lives. As you work to address the root of the problems, scenting the air around you can definitely help.

If you can scent the air while also keeping your physical environment spic-and-span, all the better! Consider the blends (and other ideas) in this chapter the next time you clean your house.

Destressing Scent

In a 2009 study, Japanese scientists found that the inhalation of linalool, a compound found in certain essential oils, such as lavender, reduced both stress levels and the activity of genes responsible for generating the chemicals associated with stress.

Other Odor-Eaters

The focus of this chapter is using essential oil diffusion to help you clean your house and get rid of unwanted odors. You will also find these other natural odor-eaters very helpful as you work to clean and enhance your environment.

Zeolite

Zeolite is a mineral known to be adsorbent to odors, meaning it actively draws odor molecules to it through its ability to absorb water, often the source of odor. Look for zeolite in pet stores — it is used to absorb pet odors and in fish tanks to filter the water.

Zeolite comes in many different forms, but is most commonly available as a powder or in granules. The smaller the particle, the greater the surface area with the capacity to absorb smells, so choose powder over granules.

As an added bonus, zeolite is reusable! Placing it in the sun will eradicate any odors it has already absorbed, meaning it can be used again and again.

As tempting as it may be to do so, do not add essential oils to zeolite. The mineral is so good at holding scents, it will sequester the oils rather than allowing them to volatilize into the air, rendering them basically useless.

Baking Soda

Like zeolite, baking soda works to absorb odors. It has the advantage of being easier to find, but seems to be somewhat less effective than zeolite. Save baking soda for lighter jobs and use zeolite for problem odors.

Clay

Clay is absorbent, but works best when dampened first. A clay paste may successfully absorb old odors from mildew stains on walls, for example. Simply make a small clay patty and place it over the stain. Once the daub has dried out, it will generally fall off on its own, and you can repeat the process as necessary.

There are many different kinds of clay; for this purpose, be sure to use white kaolin clay, which is widely available from many sources. Other clays will stain the surface a different color!

Cleaning Your Space

It is easy to clean your house using natural ingredients, which can be enhanced and scented with essential oils to strengthen the cleaning and antimicrobial effects of homemade products. With a few simple and easy-to-find ingredients, 95% of your cleaning supplies can be replaced with safer, cheaper products you can easily make at home.

The four main base materials are baking soda, distilled white vinegar, hydrogen peroxide and castile soap. Baking soda and soap can be combined to create a scrubbing cleanser, for example, and diluted vinegar cleans glass far better and faster than any commercially available cleaner. Adding hydrogen peroxide to baking soda makes a mildly bleaching paste that can quickly remove stains from grout.

There are many resources available to help you create your own cleaners, but keep in mind that any homemade cleaner will benefit from the addition of essential oils. As you clean, you will be diffusing scent into the air, helping to both freshen and clear the air, and to generally change the feel of the space.

Single Oils

- Blue chamomile
- Lavender
- Lemon
- Pine
- Rosemary
- Sweet orange

Recommended Base Soap

Dr. Bronner's liquid soap makes a good base for essential oils. Be sure to get the unscented Baby-Mild option.

Sweeter Vinegar

While it is a fantastic cleaner, let's face it: vinegar is not the yummiest smell. Sweeten it up with this blend. Use this formula wherever you would use a spray cleaner — on glass, counters, toilets and mirrors, for example.

Blend
- **Blue chamomile:** 3 drops
- **Lemon:** 3 drops
- **Lavender:** 1 to 3 drops

Cleaner
- To $\frac{1}{2}$ cup (125 mL) of white vinegar, add $1\frac{1}{2}$ cups (375 mL) of water and the oil blend.

Consider diffusing the Sweeter Vinegar blend of oils into the air as you clean, to further disguise the vinegar smell.

Scrubbing Paste

The great thing about baking soda is it is so fine, it is very unlikely to scratch any surface. Still, for safety's sake, spot-test on a hidden corner of your surface first before using this paste.

Lemon essential oil is an excellent disinfectant. In conjunction with ultraviolet rays from the sun, lemon can successfully eradicate most microbes from surfaces. Consider using the combination on your cutting board!

Blend
- **Lemon:** 3 to 5 drops
- **Sweet orange:** 1 to 3 drops
- **Rosemary or pine:** 1 drop

Cleaner
- Place $1/4$ cup (60 mL) of baking soda in a nonreactive bowl and add enough hydrogen peroxide to make a thick paste. Add the oil blend to the paste and start scrubbing immediately — this paste does not keep and will be less effective once the hydrogen peroxide and baking soda stop bubbling.

Tacky Remover

You know that sticky gum left after you peel away a price sticker? There are commercial products that will remove that irritating sticky spot, but sweet orange essential oil works like a charm! Add 1 drop to the sticky area and wait a few seconds, then rub it off with a sponge. Be sure to wash off any residual essential oil if the underlying surface is plastic or wood.

Reducing Mold and Mildew

Mold and mildew are common problems in a bathroom, especially one that is poorly ventilated (and surprisingly many are). Once a bathroom acquires a moldy smell, it is very difficult to eradicate.

Using essential oils on a mold stain can help, as many oils are antimicrobial and antifungal. It takes diligence, but consistent applications of an oil-enhanced paste (see box, below) will eventually kill off the mold.

In addition, essential oil diffusion can, with diligent use, clear a funky mildew or mold smell. Try passive diffusers that can be charged with new oil every time you visit the bathroom. A few possibilities include absorbent felt danglers, terra cotta discs or cotton balls tucked into corners.

Single Oils

- Blue chamomile
- Cinnamon
- Clary sage
- Clove
- Eucalyptus citriodora
- Eucalyptus globulus
- Eucalyptus radiata
- Lavender
- Lemon
- Lemongrass
- Myrrh
- Patchouli
- Peppermint
- Rose geranium
- Rosemary
- Thyme

Mold-Killing Paste

Add essential oils (such as the Floral Notes blend on page 186) to baking soda moistened with hydrogen peroxide to make a paste. Thickly apply this paste to the stain as often as possible. Be aware that this works by both killing the mold causing the stain and by bleaching, as the combination of baking soda and hydrogen peroxide is a lightening agent.

Spiced Apple

Blue chamomile has a fruity apple-like scent that blends well with cinnamon to create a scent reminiscent of freshly baked apple pie!

Blend
- **Blue chamomile:** 3 to 5 drops
- **Cinnamon:** 1 to 3 drops
- **Clove:** 1 drop

Diffuse
- *Passive diffuser* such as an absorbent felt dangler or a terra cotta disc.
- *Nebulizing diffuser:* Use a timer and set it to turn on for a few minutes a few times throughout the day.

If you want to add a touch of fruitiness to any oil blend, consider blue chamomile in tiny amounts.

Fresh and Bright

This blend brings a sunshine-fresh feel to a bathroom, easily counteracting that mildew or mold smell.

Blend
- **Lemon:** 8 to 10 drops
- **Eucalyptus (any type):** 3 to 5 drops
- **Rosemary:** 1 to 3 drops

Diffuse

- *Passive diffuser* such as an absorbent felt dangler or a terra cotta disc.

- *Candle-heated diffuser:* These are nice to use when company is coming, although they need monitoring to ensure that the water does not dry up.

- *Nebulizing diffuser:* No one wants to hang out in the bathroom, so use a timer to switch it off after a few minutes.

Rosemary oil's fresh, woody notes are reminiscent of a walk through an evergreen forest.

Floral Notes

This blend has the added advantage of being antifungal. Use it in Mold-Killing Paste (see box, page 185) to eradicate odor-causing fungus anywhere you find black stains on grout or tile. Diffuse these oils into the air as well, to support the antifungal properties of the paste.

Blend
- **Rose geranium:** 3 to 5 drops
- **Lavender:** 3 drops
- **Patchouli:** 1 drop

Diffuse

- *Passive diffuser* such as an absorbent felt dangler or a terra cotta disc.

- *Fan diffuser:* This has the added advantage of being a handy device to cleanse the air after visits to the toilet — flick it on as you enter, and off as you leave.

Aged patchouli is an extremely rich and aromatic oil, sweet and spicy with beautiful balsamic notes.

Dispersing Cooking Odors

The best way to get rid of old cooking smells is to use a two-pronged approach. First, use a passive absorptive substance like zeolite or baking soda (see box, page 182). Second, diffuse essential oils into the room. Because some scents can clash with leftover cooking scents, such as garlic and onion, the oils suggested here are all from plants commonly used as foods.

If you use a fan diffuser or ultrasonic diffuser, wait about 30 minutes after all cooking is completed, then run it for a few minutes to really help clear the air.

Sweet and Spicy

The scent of this blend is quite unique, but it does an excellent job of reducing cooking smells very quickly.

Blend
- **Fennel:** 3 drops
- **Cinnamon or basil:** 1 to 3 drops
- **Tarragon:** 1 drop

Diffuse
- *Stovetop diffuser:* Add the blend to about 1 inch (2.5 cm) of water in a kettle or saucepan and put it on a burner that has just been turned off, to take advantage of the radiant heat.

Dessert!

Fir has a lovely jammy fruit note that blends really well with cinnamon and vanilla. The result smells a bit like fruit pie.

Blend
- **Fir:** 3 drops (or 1 to 3 drops sweet orange)
- **Vanilla:** 3 drops
- **Cinnamon:** 1 drop

Diffuse
- *Scented wax warmer:* Make a wax form (see page 23) with a few drops of this blend. If you are using an unscented wax form and adding the scent at the time of use, add the oil blend after the wax has melted.

Single Oils
- Anise
- Basil
- Cinnamon
- Clove
- Fennel
- Fir
- Grapefruit
- Lemon
- Lemongrass
- Peppermint
- Red mandarin
- Rosemary
- Sweet orange
- Tarragon
- Vanilla

Stovetop diffusion can also help divert excess heat from the stovetop that would have gone into further heating up the kitchen.

You can substitute 8 to 10 drops of high-quality vanilla extract for the vanilla essential oil in the Dessert! blend.

Citrus Fresh

Citrus scent is a natural in the kitchen!

Blend

- **Grapefruit:** 1 drop
- **Lemon:** 1 drop
- **Sweet orange:** 1 drop

Diffuse

- *Passive diffusers:* These work well here, as citrus scents are quite strong but somewhat fugitive (they dissipate quickly). Allowing the scent to diffuse passively means it will stick around much longer!

- *Fan diffuser:* If you are looking for a quick blast of scent instead of a lingering one, consider running a fan diffuser for a few minutes. Be sure to wait about 30 minutes after completing the cooking.

Grapefruit oil is incredibly fresh and uplifting, without being overwhelming. The scent is fresh and intensely citrusy, with a sweet undertone. Some people detect bitter notes as well.

Bright and Light

The bright, light scents of the oils in this blend help eradicate the stagnant, heavy smells left after cooking, bringing fresh energy back to the space.

Blend

- **Sweet orange:** 3 to 5 drops
- **Basil:** 1 drop
- **Peppermint:** 1 drop

Diffuse

- *Stovetop diffuser:* Add the blend to a small pot of water on the stove after you prepare a meal. It makes use of the residual heat from a burner quite nicely!

- *Passive diffuser:* Place a passive diffuser in a sunny window so you can enjoy the aroma as you cook, and to clear odors after cooking.

Peppermint wakes up the nose, and basil grounds the scent. Sweet orange supports them both with its happy, bright scent.

Banishing Musty Odors

Musty smells in a laundry room kind of defeat the purpose of cleaning our clothes and linens. Especially in the winter, many people find they have to dry their laundry inside, and musty odors easily impregnate the clothes as they dry. Keep your clothes smelling fresh and clean with the oils listed here.

It will probably not be enough to run a diffuser in the laundry room or basement for a few minutes at a time. Instead, a passive diffuser regularly charged up with fresh oils is a good way to go. Try hanging a few absorbent felt danglers near the dryer vent. If you are also using an odor-absorbing substance, such as zeolite or baking soda (see box, page 182), be sure to place it on the other side of the room so the oils do not get absorbed right away!

Single Oils

- Basil
- Eucalyptus citriodora
- Fir
- Grapefruit
- Lavender
- Lemon
- Lemongrass
- Oakmoss
- Peppermint
- Pine
- Rosemary
- Spruce
- Tea tree
- Thyme linalool

Homemade Dryer Sheets

Try scenting your clothes with homemade dryer sheets. Cut out small sheets of wool felt and add a few drops of your favorite oil. Wool has the added advantage of acting as a fabric softener.

Clean and Fresh

This blend is both fresh and antimicrobial, and may help reduce the cause of musty odors — namely, damp and mold.

Blend
- **Grapefruit:** 5 to 8 drops
- **Eucalyptus citriodora:** 3 to 5 drops
- **Thyme linalool:** 1 drop

Diffuse
- *Smelling salts:* Add the blend to a small container of salt and leave it open to the air at all times. The salt will have to be changed out frequently, as it will also absorb ambient moisture — another benefit!

In addition to being citrus-like, the scent of eucalyptus citriodora oil is somewhat rosy, with a slightly balsamic finish.

Forest Floor

There may be no scents more clean-smelling than the evergreens. This blend is guaranteed to freshen a space and reduce musty odors.

Blend

- **Pine:** 5 to 8 drops
- **Rosemary:** 3 to 5 drops
- **Oakmoss:** 1 drop

Diffuse

- *Passive diffuser:* If there is a window in your laundry room or basement, consider placing terra cotta discs on the sill to passively diffuse whenever the sun is out. While they will diffuse on a cloudy day, they really shine when the sun does. These can also be used quite easily in conjunction with other diffusers.

Add 1 or 2 drops of the Forest Floor blend to the water you use to clean — in a mop bucket, for example. A few drops, even spread over a large area, will still be subtly detectable.

Evicting Unwanted Houseguests

So many critters just love taking over the attic. I guess it makes sense: it's dark, warm and protected, with a handy little vent like a doorway just asking them to come inside. While I love being hospitable, they do tend to do a fair bit of damage — chewing wires, stealing insulation, leaving deposits of various kinds…

It is definitely extra work to diffuse essential oils in the attic, a space we do not typically enter often. If you have an animal, insect or bird infestation, though, diffusing can really help drive them out, letting you take back your home. The great thing about essential oils used in this way is that they are not toxic, so they will not kill or injure the invaders but will simply make the space less inviting to them.

All of the oils listed here work so well that any blend you want to create will probably work. Consider using the last drips from any nearly empty bottle! For that matter, I often open up empty bottles and place them in the attic or basement — just be sure to leave the plastic restrictor cap as well, as it is usually covered in essential oil even after the bottle is long empty.

Some oils have a good track record against certain unwelcome guests. See the suggested blends below for more help with specific invasions.

Single Oils

- Basil
- Bay laurel
- Bergamot
- Cedarwood
- Cinnamon
- Clove
- Cypress
- Eucalyptus citriodora
- Eucalyptus globulus
- Hyssop decumbens
- Lavender
- Lemongrass
- Peppermint
- Pine
- Sweet orange
- Tea tree

Attic Vents

Those wide-open vents really do need to be addressed if you want the critters to get out and stay out. While they cannot be blocked (obviously), if they are not already screened, do so as soon as possible. Also consider using some of the whole plant materials that produce the essential oils in this list: stack them between two layers of screening — a wider mesh, a fairly thin layer of plant material, then a finer mesh — and place it in front of the vent. This definitely helped in my house.

Mice

While these little critters are hard to spot, you can usually tell there is an infestation from signs like chewed paper or droppings. There is often a distinctive smell, as well.

Blend
- **Eucalyptus citriodora:** 8 to 10 drops
- **Peppermint:** 3 to 5 drops
- **Bergamot:** 1 to 3 drops

Diffuse

- *Fan diffuser:* Consider putting the diffuser on a timer set to turn on for a few minutes several times throughout the night, when mice are most active.

- *Cotton balls:* Saturate several cotton balls with the blend and place them near where you suspect the mice might be getting in.

Avoid touching sensitive tissues, like your eyes, after preparing a cotton ball — it's best to wash your hands immediately, just in case.

Bird Repellent

Birds apparently don't like garlic. If you have birds nesting in your attic (or anywhere you don't want them, like window ledges), you can create your own garlic oil by making a paste of garlic and covering it with oil (for use as a pest repellent, it doesn't really matter what oil you choose). Some recipes suggest adding cayenne pepper at this point. Let the oil sit in a dark space for a few days, shaking at least once daily. Remove the garlic by pressing the oil through cheesecloth. The oil can now be added to cotton balls or pads and placed wherever you would prefer the birds not to be. Don't forget to reuse the cheesecloth for this purpose as well — you will never be able to use it for anything else, after all!

Some folks add the garlic oil to a bit of apple cider vinegar and water in a spritzer. If you choose this method, remember to shake well to blend. Vinegar and oil, after all …

Flies and Mosquitoes

No one likes these unwelcome guests! Fortunately, these pests are very sensitive to strong scents and are easily driven off by diffusion. Remember to bring your diffuser outside with you when you relax on the deck.

Blend
- **Basil:** 3 to 5 drops
- **Lemongrass:** 3 to 5 drops (or 1 to 3 drops eucalyptus citriodora)
- **Clove:** 1 drop

Diffuse

- *Passive diffusers:* Felt danglers work well, especially if the problem is outside, as small breezes will help disperse the scent.

- *Ultrasonic* or *nebulizing diffuser:* Because flies and mosquitoes tend to be summertime woes, these diffusers are a good choice, as they will disperse the essential oils without heating the house.

- *Spritzer:* Add the entire blend to distilled water and keep the spritzer nearby when dining al fresco. Be sure to place it in a cool, shady spot, as heat and sun will cause the essential oils to deteriorate more quickly. Remember, shake well before spritzing into the air around your picnic table or blanket.

Instead of using clove essential oil, try soaking whole cloves in the basil and lemongrass oils. Place the dish in a prominent place near the problem and watch those flies fly away!

Citronella

So many references suggest citronella to address pest problems, but citronella can be harsh, and some people (including yours truly) find it downright offensive. Fortunately, its active ingredients — citronellol, citronellal and geraniol — are found in many essential oils that have a much more enticing aroma. Why not try lemongrass, rose geranium or rose instead? On the other hand, if you like the smell of citronella, it is usually relatively cheap, so by all means use it!

Cockroaches

Despite cockroaches' reputation for being impossible to eradicate, this blend is surprisingly effective! Be sure to spray everywhere you suspect the roaches are entering your house, and regularly diffuse in the same areas.

Blend

- **Peppermint:** 10 drops
- **Cypress:** 5 to 8 drops
- **Hyssop decumbens:** 3 to 5 drops

Diffuse

- *Spritzer:* Add at least 10 drops of the blend to a spritzer with some tap water. Shake well before spritzing.

- *Fan* or *nebulizing diffuser:* Add a timer to the diffuser, set to come on for a few minutes several times overnight, when roaches are most active.

It is important to note that no other variety of hyssop is either safe or effective, so be sure to buy only essential oil made from *Hyssop officinalis* var. *decumbens.*

Ants

These clever critters can crawl through the smallest cracks to invade your space. Fortunately, essential oil diffusion works really well to drive them away.

Blend
- **Tea tree:** 3 to 5 drops
- **Bay laurel:** 1 to 3 drops
- **Cinnamon:** 1 drop

Diffuse

Always protect the surfaces cotton balls are placed on, as there is nothing stopping the oils from seeping through the cotton and staining the underlying area.

- *Cotton balls:* Saturate several cotton balls with the blend and place them near where you suspect the ants might be getting in.

- *Smelling salts:* Add the blend to salt and stir well. Place a small piece of paper where you suspect the ants are getting in and scatter the salt over the paper to disrupt their scent trail.

- *Spritzer:* Add to a spritzer bottle filled with water for "spot treatments." While I truly dislike killing anything, it is a fact that the fewer the number of ants that return to the nest, the fewer "maps" the rest of the colony receives. So spritz away and watch those critters scatter!

Cracks

If bugs are getting into your house through cracks, essential oils or blends can be dripped directly into the gaps. Keep in mind that discoloration may occur, so be careful not to drip oils on any surface you want to maintain. The whole herbs that make the oils can be used in this way, too — I stick whole bay laurel leaves under my windowsill, where ants get in, and it stops them in their tracks.

Destressing Your Space

In "Environmental Health Is Personal Health" (page 181), I discussed how important it is to reduce stress and distress whenever possible, to help you stay as healthy as possible. When you need to destress, you can use any essential oil that helps you feel great! The suggestions here are some single oils and blends known to help with specific stressors, like fatigue or road drama. Many of the blends recommended in "Improving Your Health with Essential Oils" (pages 80–180) address specific stressors, so be sure to check out those sections as well!

Work Space Mood Booster

Whether we like it or not, most jobs expect us to remain actively engaged for 8 long hours, despite the natural ebb and flow of interest we all experience throughout the day. This blend will help wake up the mind, energize the body and improve the mood so you can stay on point.

Blend
- **Lemon:** 5 to 8 drops
- **Black spruce:** 1 to 3 drops
- **Rosemary:** 1 to 3 drops

Diffuse
- *Nebulizing or passive diffuser:* Use a nebulizing diffuser if allowed by your workplace, or use a passive diffuser to limit the reach of the scent to just your work area.

- *Personal diffuser:* If you cannot diffuse into your work space because you share it with others, carry a small personal diffuser, like smelling salts, that will lightly scent your area and can be sniffed for a stronger effect if needed.

Black spruce has a fruity undertone, but is primarily balsamic and bright. It is an incredibly uplifting scent, and is used in formulas to increase energy and circulation.

Auto Mood Booster

If there's anyplace you absolutely need a pleasant, unstressful environment, it's when you are driving, especially if you drive in traffic every day. This blend is calming and increases alertness.

Blend
- **Eucalyptus (any type):** 3 to 5 drops
- **Cinnamon:** 1 drop
- **Peppermint:** 1 drop

Diffuse
- *Car plug-in diffuser:* The obvious choice here, but a good one.
- *Smelling salts:* Place a tin of smelling salts with a perforated lid in your car, allowing the essential oil molecules to waft out as you drive.
- *Terra cotta disc:* This is what I use in my car. I added a little nonslip pad to my dashboard to keep it in place. Be sure to remove it if you park in the sun, or the residual oils may leave an off-smell in the car.

If using a car plug-in diffuser, do not run it for too long, or the heat may corrupt the oils.

Clearing Your House by Burning Plants

These days, we tend to default to the easiest way, and adding a drop or two of oil to a diffuser is far easier than burning plant material. On the other hand, the long tradition of using dried plants to scent the house deserves at least a mention. Besides, the odor left in a house from fragrant smoke is far richer and more complex than that left by essential oils. Nothing matches the coumarin-rich fragrance of burning sweetgrass, for example, or the dense, heady scent of melting frankincense resin.

Be sure to take all the precautions necessary to avoid damage to surfaces when burning, well, anything!

The plants listed here are just a sampling. If you are interested in "smudging" (one of the names given to this practice), there are many books available on the subject. See the Resources (page 207) for some recommendations.

- **Cedar:** Cedar smoke is clarifying and refreshing, while also helping with focus. Like the essential oil, cedar smoke can strengthen endurance, and cedar is traditionally burned in sweat lodge and other Native American ceremonies for this purpose.

- **Copal:** Widely used in Mexico and in Central and South America, copal is a resin gathered from a species of tree used medicinally where it grows. Copal smoke can clear the mind when the intention is to focus on the infinite, not the day to day, and is utilized to deepen meditation practices.

- **Frankincense and myrrh:** These two resins are frequently used together and, even if burned individually, offer many of the same benefits. They are used in many Christian traditions to raise awareness to heaven and carry prayers to God. Both are somewhat earthy, so they also help keep us grounded in the spiritual experience, so to speak.

- **Sage:** Sage bundles have been used by Native Americans for centuries in clearing rituals designed to remove negative influences from the immediate environment. The scent of burning sage is savory and dense — some find it overwhelming. If you are interested in ritually clearing negative energy, consider sage.

- **Sandalwood:** The sandalwood tree is endangered, so be sure to obtain the wood only from ethically harvested trees. Very popular in both ancient and modern times, the scent of sandalwood is nearly ubiquitous in temples throughout Asia and on altars around the world. It is said to center one's attention and may help open the third eye, associated with intuition and messages from guides.

- **Sweetgrass:** Sweetgrass is commonly used to invite in positive energy. It reminds me of the scent of a field of hay on a very sunny day — the light, happy, sweet smell of this burning grass is uplifting. Many people will follow a sage smudge with a bit of burning sweetgrass.

Appendix 1:

Base Oils for Topical Treatments

Therapeutic Properties

In addition to being a foundation for the essential oils, acting to dilute them to a safe percentage for topical application, base oils add therapeutic properties to the blends. Many base oils are high in absorbable vitamins or cofactors, and some have special protective properties.

Although this book is primarily about diffusing essential oils to help with health imbalances, in many places I have suggested adding an essential oil blend to a base oil for use as a topical application to support the benefits of diffusion.

The choice of an appropriate base oil depends on many factors, including the desired viscosity, how the oil feels on the skin and especially the blend's intended use. If the treatment needs to absorb rapidly into the bloodstream, the oil should be unsaturated — as most oils from fruits, nuts and seeds are. The main exception is coconut oil, which contains a type of saturated fat. Saturated fats help to keep the treatment on the skin longer, so they may be more effective when treating skin conditions, for example.

Research Roundup

There have been some interesting studies showing that transdermal (across the skin) absorption of gross nutrients does happen — as unlikely as that would seem, given the nature of the skin as a protective barrier. In 1974, an article published in *The Lancet*, the U.K.'s premier medical journal, reported on essential fatty acid deficiencies being successfully treated with topical applications of sunflower oil. Still, generally speaking, the molecular weight of most base oils is too high to be absorbed transdermally. For our purposes, we are mainly interested in base oils known for their ability to hold essential oil molecules in place so that they can be more slowly absorbed into the bloodstream or, for skin conditions, so that they can be used as treatment at the site of application.

Argan Oil *(Argania spinosa)*

Grown primarily in Morocco, argan oil is also commonly known as Morocco oil. Argan oil production relies on the traditional process of harvesting the seeds: goats eat the fruit but leave the seeds, which are collected later by the farmers. Argan oil production is a very old tradition in Morocco, and is still important to the economy of the region.

The seeds must be roasted and cracked to release the oil, but the oil is mechanically cold-pressed without heat. It is an excellent emollient oil — it is high in antioxidants and vitamin E, making it perfect for reducing free radicals at the surface. It also helps stabilize oil blends. Argan is known for its skin-strengthening properties and is especially wonderful for increasing elasticity.

Avocado Oil *(Persea americana)*

Fruit fats are quite rare, so take advantage of this wonderful source, cold-pressed from the dehydrated flesh of the avocado. Avocados contain high levels of fat-soluble vitamin A and vitamin D, so the oil oxidizes more slowly. (Many fats from plants native to hot climates have this quality.) Avocado oil is also high in lecithin, often used as an emulsifier to keep ingredients from separating.

> **Did You Know?**
>
> Like olive and sesame oil, avocado oil is somewhat protective against damage from ultraviolet rays.

Borage Oil *(Borago officinalis)*

Bees love borage, a beautiful annual that readily self-seeds, so it is an excellent choice for a garden. The oil, cold-pressed from borage seeds, is good for dry, aging skin, both when taken internally and when applied topically. It is an excellent choice for postmenopausal women, as it is high in gamma-linolenic acid (GLA), which becomes harder for the body to synthesize as we age.

Coconut Oil *(Cocos nucifera)*

Therapeutic coconut oil is cold-pressed from the copra (blended water and flesh from inside the nut). Coconut oil is one of the few nonanimal saturated fats. The benefit of saturated oils is they "lock" therapeutic ingredients in place wherever the blend is applied, delivering the medicinal benefits slowly over time. Saturated fats are also much less likely to go rancid, so adding a bit of coconut oil to a blend may extend its shelf life. Coconut oil is very lubricating and, like many oils, has some antimicrobial benefits. It is commonly used in the production of soap.

> **Did You Know?**
>
> In earlier times, goose grease blended with herbs was used as a chest rub — coconut oil is a much nicer way to achieve the same results.

Evening Primrose Oil
(Oenothera spp.)

Evening primrose oil is an excellent choice to help with hormonal balance in conditions like premenstrual syndrome or to address symptoms of menopause. To use as a treatment for eczema, pierce a gel cap and add a few drops to an essential oil blend, then apply directly to the lesions. Do not use for too long, however — no more than a few weeks to a month.

Hazelnut Oil *(Corylus avellana)*

Cold-pressed from the hazelnut, this oil is somewhat astringent and may help with oily or boggy tissues. It is thought to increase circulation, which further helps with these issues. Plus, it has a less greasy feel than most other base oils.

A Word of Caution

Hempseed oil may have blood-thinning properties, so use it with caution if you are on medication that also thins the blood.

Hempseed Oil *(Cannabis sativa)*

Hemp seeds are remarkably rich in gamma-linolenic acid (GLA), and the greatest benefits are gained when the seeds or oil are ingested. Taken internally, the oil helps with eczema and psoriasis, and in my clinical experience, topical applications can also help these conditions. Be sure to purchase organic hempseed oil, as this is the only option produced by cold-pressing the seeds. Nonorganic hempseed oil is removed by solvents.

Did You Know?

Jojoba oil is very similar in chemical structure to human sebum, and the skin, even in sensitive individuals, typically receives it well.

Jojoba Oil *(Simmondsia chinensis)*

The jojoba plant is indigenous to the southwestern United States. The "oil," mechanically expressed from the seeds, is actually a rather rare substance: a liquid composed of wax esters, primarily made up of long-chain fatty acids and long-chain fatty alcohols. Len Price, who literally wrote the book on base oils (see Resources, page 206), reports: "There is some evidence that jojoba wax, despite consisting mainly of saturated fatty acids, can permeate the skin ... it appears to moisturize and soften the skin."

Jojoba seems to have sebum-dissolving properties, so it is an excellent choice for skin conditions like acne. Moreover, studies show that many common strains of bacteria will not grow in jojoba, making it even more appropriate for acne. Similarly, because the candida fungus cannot grow in jojoba oil, it is a useful addition to suppositories.

Jojoba oil has phenomenal oxidative stability, meaning it does not become rancid like other oils. I have kept a properly stored bottle for upward of 10 years with no perceptible change — yet another reason it makes an excellent base oil.

Macadamia Nut Oil
(Macadamia ternifolia)

Cold-pressed from the nuts of the macadamia tree, which are remarkably rich in oil, macadamia nut oil is high in palmitoleic acid, also found in high concentration in the sebum of young children. For this reason, consider it for aging skin. It has a reputation for being easily absorbed into the skin without leaving a greasy residue, so it's a good choice for those who are put off by the idea of applying oil to the skin.

Olive Oil (Olea europaea)

Most people have olive oil in their pantry, and it is an excellent medicine that has been used for thousands of years. In the baths of Ancient Rome, olive oil was used as a cleanser — the oil was slathered onto the body, then scraped off with a strigil, a tool reserved for this purpose. Today, in Greece and other countries that produce the oil, it is still a common practice to use olive oil as a lubricant for the skin and hair. The oil is mechanically extracted from the fermented fruits. The first pressing, labeled "extra virgin olive oil," is the most therapeutic.

Did You Know?

A blend of olive, sesame and avocado oils provides a small amount of protection from ultraviolet rays, although it should not be relied upon to prevent sunburn.

Rosehip Oil (Rosa rugosa or Rosa spp.)

Rosehip oil is extracted from the fruit and seeds of the rose plant. Because it is very high in vitamin C, known to help encourage healing of the skin, rosehip oil has a remarkable ability to help wounds heal without scarring. Be sure to purchase organic oil, as a lot of rosehip oil is extracted with solvents.

Sea Buckthorn Oil
(Hippophae rhamnoides)

Unlike most of the base oils discussed here, sea buckthorn oil is not expressed; rather, it is obtained by macerating sea buckthorn fruit into another oil, such as almond or olive oil. The resulting oil is high in essential fatty acids, which are beneficial to the skin. Consider sea buckthorn oil for treating rosacea or skin ulcerations.

Sesame Oil (Sesamum indicum)

The sesame plant has been cultivated for thousands of years and is grown all over the world; many cultures rely on the seeds for their cuisine. The oil, pressed from the seeds, is somewhat protective against damage from ultraviolet rays. It

Did You Know?

Like most nuts and seeds, sesame seeds are high in calcium and magnesium, minerals that can help build bone strength and reduce muscle cramps.

is one of the most commonly used oils in Ayurvedic medicine, employed primarily for its warming property — it is an excellent massage component whenever one has been exposed to cold. Sesame oil contains antioxidants, so it has a long shelf life if stored appropriately.

Sunflower Oil *(Helianthus annuus)*

Sunflower oil is one of my favorites to use as a base, as it is slightly warming and moves stagnant fluids, making it useful for any imbalance of stagnation, like edema. According to Len Price, the author of *Carrier Oils for Aromatherapy and Massage*, it may also be helpful for asthma. Be sure to purchase organic sunflower oil, as this is the only option produced by cold-pressing the seeds. Nonorganic sunflower oil is removed by solvents.

Sweet Almond Oil
(Prunus dulcis)

While it is less likely to become rancid — a real bonus — sweet almond oil is more oily-feeling than others, making it less desirable to some people. It is a common addition to many topical preparations and massage blends. Be sure to purchase only organic cold-pressed almond oil.

Tamanu Oil
(Calophyllum inophyllum)

The *Calophyllum inophyllum* tree is native to many islands in the Indian Ocean and South Pacific and has a different name everywhere it grows — you might find it as *foraha* (Madagascar), *fetau* (Samoa) or *kamani* (Hawaii). A lot of *Calophyllum inophyllum* oil comes from Tahiti, where it is called *tamanu*. Tamanu is a bit of a "medicine chest in a bottle" for the people of these islands, used for many different kinds of complaints, from diaper rash and bug bites to vitiligo and leprosy. Tamanu oil is cold-pressed from the fruit after it has been sun-dried for at least several weeks. It is particularly helpful against neuralgic pain from shingles and is anti-inflammatory and nonirritating to mucous membranes.

No Fear of Allergies

Oils pressed from nuts are not generally triggers for those with allergies, likely because protein, the component considered to be the most suspect allergy-triggering agent, is absent from refined oils.

Appendix 2:
Using Essential Oils for Immune Support and Detox

Immune Support

In my opinion, the human immune system is deeply underappreciated. Not only does it work nonstop to keep potential invaders from accessing the body through the skin and other entry points, but it must also assess every substance that does make it in and decide whether it is a threat. Even nutrients from the food we eat are assessed by the immune system before we can use them! This evaluation happens in the liver, an organ that has a huge role in keeping invaders out of the blood.

Which brings us to an interesting point: unlike the digestive or circulatory system, the immune system isn't really a "system" on its own; rather, it is a part of every other system in the body. The best way to support the immune system is to ensure that we take the best care of ourselves we can, at every level, by avoiding substances that tax the body, like processed foods or alcohol, and by exercising regularly to keep the blood moving — blood carries many immune factors that must constantly circulate throughout the body as our first line of internal defense.

In these modern times of increased synthetics, the immune system has to work extra-hard as it encounters substances that are not natural and are therefore difficult to assess. As a result, the immune system can become hypervigilant and attack substances that are not, in fact, harmful, like our own tissues. Autoimmune diseases, which can wreak havoc on the human body, are the result of an overactive immune system, and if you are suffering from one, boosting your immune system is the last thing you want to do!

Dry Skin Brushing

Try dry skin brushing for immune support. This amazingly effective technique encourages movement through the lymphatic system, to keep it healthy. For more information, see the box on page 139.

Fortunately, many essential oils are bidirectional, or balancing, meaning they help the body return to a healthy state of homeodynamics — but not for everyone! If you suffer from an autoimmune disorder, it really is best to work very closely with a trained professional and avoid treating yourself at home.

For the rest of us, the Stay Healthy Blend (see box, below) can help boost the immune system during cold and flu season, to help us stay healthy when everyone around us is coughing up infectious agents into the air we breathe.

Stay Healthy Blend

This is a great blend to use with a nebulizing diffuser anywhere those suffering from a cold or flu have been. I use it in my treatment rooms during cold and flu season. Diffuse for a few minutes several times a day to reduce the microbial load and enhance and strengthen your immune system.

- Eucalyptus globulus or tea tree: 5 to 8 drops
- Lavender: 5 to 8 drops
- Lemon: 1 drop

Detoxification

Use Natural Beauty Products

Avoiding beauty products packed with synthetic ingredients will also reduce the burden on many organs, including the skin. Look for natural products that use essential oils, or make your own! This is a very enjoyable way to add the benefits of aromatherapy to your routine.

A final word regarding the use of essential oils to aid in detoxification. In keeping with the ideas laid out above, it should be clear that treating your body well is the best way to detoxify. The main organs that eliminate toxins are the digestive system and the liver, but the kidneys, the skin and the lungs are also constantly sweeping substances out of the body. Keeping these organs in tiptop shape allows them to do their job efficiently. You can reduce the liver's burden by avoiding alcohol, for example, or support the lungs by quitting smoking. Reducing your intake of toxins is the best way to remove toxins from your body.

Lately, some companies have started to promote the internal use of essential oils to support the body in its natural functions of removing unwanted substances. However, since the liver automatically marks anything that enters our body as an "invader," the increased burden of ingested essential oils on the liver may entirely negate any benefits the oils are purported to offer.

In my opinion, it is a much better idea to support your detoxification organs by eating healthy food, exercising and avoiding substances that add to the burden of their work. If these organs become unbalanced, using essential oils to support them might make sense, but use those essential oils in a diffuser.

Acknowledgments

Writing a book is always a joint project, as all the teachers I have ever encountered are embedded in the words I write. By teachers, I do not just mean the educators in front of whom I have sat for countless hours — though they are, of course, responsible for some of the knowledge I share here. The teachers I mean are the people who taught me what it is to live a good life, in alignment with my true nature, according to principles worth sharing. These principles may not be explicitly stated in the text (although many are), but they shape my every action so must be reflected in the material. I thank you here, as I did not when you gave me your gifts, for they usually sent me deep into thought as I watched my paradigm shift and grow.

I have spent the last several years writing books, healing and growing into a new understanding of life. I have been supported in this by good friends, many of whom I met through social media before meeting them in person. I admit to having some doubts, when I first encountered social media, about their power for good and constructive growth. But when my life was turned upside down by one particular wave of shocks, I turned to social media to describe the experience. The responses I received from people all over the world helped me in ways I could never have imagined. The connections felt tenuous at first, but the strength and encouragement I received from these erstwhile strangers radically transformed my perspective as our connection grew. I recently traveled for an extended period (six months, on and off) and met many of these online friends. The reality of them was, in every case, even more wonderful than their online presence had led me to believe. It was an awakening, and has profoundly recreated who I am. I am so grateful to these new friends for their support.

Specifically, I must once again thank the CoDB group for supporting me as we rode the waves of sorrow and joy together. In particular, I want to thank my dear friend Monika Sovine for helping me return to life at a time when I felt like retreating into a cave, away from the world and the suffering of so many. Your boundless enthusiasm for living and experiencing beauty reminded me of how life can be lived, is supposed to be lived. I love you with all my heart, Minks, and will be forever grateful for your generous spirit.

Resources

Further Reading

Aromatherapy

Aftel, Mandy. *Fragrant: The Secret Life of Scent.* Warwickshire: Riverhead Books, 2014.

Arctander, Steffen. *Perfume and Flavor Materials of Natural Origin.* Elizabeth, NJ: 1960.

Franchomme, Pierre, Roger Jollois and Daniel Pénoël. *L'aromathérapie exactement: Encyclopédie de l'utilisation thérapeutique des huiles essentielles.* Montreal: Roger Jollois, 1990.

Keville, Kathi, and Mindy Green. *Aromatherapy: A Complete Guide to the Healing Art,* 2nd edition. Feasterville Trevose, PA: Crossing Press, 2008.

Mojay, Gabriel. *Aromatherapy for Healing the Spirit: Restoring Emotional and Mental Balance with Essential Oils.* Rochester, VT: Healing Arts Press, 2000.

Price, Shirley, and Len Price, eds. *Aromatherapy for Health Professionals,* 4th edition. London: Churchill Livingstone, 2011.

Schnaubelt, Kurt. *Advanced Aromatherapy: The Science of Essential Oil Therapy.* Rochester, VT: Healing Arts Press, 1998.

Tisserand, Robert, and Rodney Young. *Essential Oil Safety: A Guide for Health Care Professionals,* 2nd edition. London: Churchill Livingstone, 2013.

Herbal Medicine

Hoffmann, David. *Medical Herbalism: The Science and Practice of Herbal Medicine.* Rochester, VT: Healing Arts Press, 2003.

Tilgner, Sharol Marie. *Herbal Medicine from the Heart of the Earth,* 2nd edition. Pleasant Hill, OR: Wise Acres, 2009.

History of Scent and Scent Materials

Aftel, Mandy. *Essence and Alchemy: A Natural History of Perfume.* Layton, UT: Gibbs Smith, 2004.

Classen, Constance, David Howes and Anthony Synnott. *Aroma: The Cultural History of Smell.* London: Routledge, 1994.

Reinarz, Jonathan. *Past Scents: Historical Perspectives on Smell.* Champaign, IL: University of Illinois Press, 2014.

Turin, Luca. *The Secret of Scent: Adventures in Perfume and the Science of Smell.* New York: Harper Perennial, 2007.

Base Oils

Price, Len, with Shirley Price. *Carrier Oils: For Aromatherapy and Massage,* 4th edition. Warwickshire: Riverhead Books, 2000.

Supply Sources

Hydrosols

Catty, Suzanne. *Hydrosols: The Next Aromatherapy.* Rochester, VT: Healing Arts Press, 2001.

Harman, Ann. *Harvest to Hydrosol: Distill Your Own Exquisite Hydrosols at Home.* Fruitland, WA: botANNicals, 2015.

Incense

Toy, Barbara. *Traveling the Incense Route: From Arabia to the Levant in the Footsteps of the Magi.* New York: Tauris Parke Paperbacks, 2009.

Wylundt and Steven R. Smith. *Wylundt's Book of Incense.* Newburyport, MA: Red Wheel/Weiser, 2007.

Smudging

Donatella, LeeZa. *Smudging for Beginners: Secrets from a Professional.* Park City, UT: Higher Roads Productions, 2015.

Ronngren, Diane. *Sage & Smudge: The Ultimate Guide.* Carlsbad, CA: ETC Publishing, 2003.

Bottles

Bulk Apothecary
www.bulkapothecary.com

Specialty Bottle
www.specialtybottle.com

Base Materials

Essential Wholesale & Labs
www.essentialwholesale.com/category/32/ingredients

Blotter Paper for Danglers

Candles & Supplies
www.candlesandsupplies.net/Air-Fresheners/Air-Freshener-Paper

Inhalation Sticks

Amazon
www.amazon.com (Search: personal inhaler essential oils)

References

American Chemical Society. Stop and smell the flowers — the scent really can soothe stress. *ScienceDaily*, 2009 Jul 23. Available at: www.sciencedaily.com/releases/2009/07/090722110901.htm.

Anonymous. *The Classic of Mountains and Seas*. Translated by Anne Birrell. London: Penguin Classics, 2000.

Bearden M. Sharyn Gildea: Making rosaries from flowers. *U.S. Catholic*, 2010 Feb; 75 (2); 24–28.

BibleVerseStudy.com. Spikenard. Available at: www.bibleversestudy.com/johngospel/john12-spikenard-bethany.htm.

Chervinskaya AV, Zilber NA. Halotherapy for treatment of respiratory diseases. *J Aerosol Med*, 1995; 8 (3): 221–32.

China Daily. Ancient incense craze. Available at: www.chinadaily.com.cn/ezine/2007-05/18/content_875434.htm.

Choi SY, Park K. Effect of inhalation of aromatherapy oil on patients with perennial allergic rhinitis: A randomized controlled trial. *Evid Based Complement Alternat Med*, 2016; 2016: 7896081.

Edwards-Jones V, Buck R, Shawcross SG, et al. The effect of essential oils on methicillin-resistant *Staphylococcus aureus* using a dressing model. *Burns*, 2004 Dec; 30 (8): 772–77.

Hajar R. The air of history (part II): Medicine in the Middle Ages. *Heart Views*, 2012 Oct–Dec; 13 (4): 158–62.

Harissis HV. A bittersweet story: The true nature of the laurel of the Oracle of Delphi. *Perspect Biol Med*, 2014 Summer; 57 (3): 351–60.

Ibn-Sina H. *Canon of Medicine: Book II Materia Medica* (English translation of the critical Arabic text). New Delhi: Department of Islamic Studies, Hamdard University, 1998.

Lv XN, Liu ZJ, Zhang HJ, Tzeng CM. Aromatherapy and the central nerve system (CNS): Therapeutic mechanism and its associated genes. *Curr Drug Targets*, 2013 Jul; 14 (8): 872–79.

Lyttelton C. *The Scent Trail: How One Woman's Quest for the Perfect Perfume Took Her Around the World*. London: Penguin Publishing Group, 2009.

Mahe Y. History of gloves and their significance: Part I – early fashion gloves. *Fashion Times*, 2013 Nov 12. Available at: www.fashionintime.org/history-gloves-significance.

Nadel D, Danin A, Power RC, et al. Earliest floral grave lining from 13,700–11,700-y-old Natufian burials at Raqefet Cave, Mt. Carmel, Israel. *PNAS*, 2013 May; 110 (29): 11774–78.

Native Americans Online. The purification ceremony. Available at: www.native-americans-online.com/native-american-sweat-lodge.html.

Panda H. *The Complete Technology Book on Herbal Perfumes and Cosmetics*. Delhi: National Institute of Industrial Research, 2003.

Pauli A, Schilcher H. Specific selection of essential oil compounds for treatment of children's infection diseases. *Pharmaceuticals* (Basel), 2004 Jan; 1 (1): 1–30.

Pliny the Elder. *Natural History*, book XXV, chapter 19.

Poon A. The orchid and Confucius. *Asia Sentinel*, 2008 Feb 6. Available at: www.asiasentinel.com/alice-poon/culture/the-orchid-and-confucius.

Press M, Hartop PJ, Prottey C. Correction of essential fatty-acid deficiency in man by the cutaneous application of sunflower-seed oil. *Lancet*, 1974 Apr 6; 1 (7858): 597–98.

Price L. *Carrier Oils: For Aromatherapy and Massage*, 4th ed. Warwickshire: Riverhead Books, 2008.

Pybus DH, Sell CS. *The Chemistry of Fragrances*. London: Royal Society of Chemistry, 1999.

Scentcillo. Scenting places and spaces in Chinese culture. Available at: www.scentcillo.com/blog/scenting-places-and-spaces-chinese-culture.

Schnaubelt K. *Advanced Aromatherapy: The Science of Essential Oil Therapy*. Rochester, VT: Healing Arts Press, 1998.

Shaath NA. The wonders of jojoba. *happi*, 2012 Sep: 47–52.

SWCS Media. Money in the New Testament. Available at: www.swcs.com.au/moneynt.htm.

von Bingen H. *Hildegard's Healing Plants: From Her Medieval Classic Physica*. Translated by Bruce W. Hozeski. Boston: Beacon Press, 2001.

Walton G. Patchouli in the 1800s. Geri Walton: Unique Histories from the 18th and 19th Centuries. Available at: www.geriwalton.com/patchouli.

Williamson AM, Feyer A-M. Moderate sleep deprivation produces impairments in cognitive and motor performance equivalent to legally prescribed levels of alcohol intoxication. *Occup Environ Med*, 2000; 57: 649–55.

Yang S. *The Divine Farmer's Materia Medica: A Translation of the Shen Nong Ben Cao Jing*. Boulder: Blue Poppy Press, 1998.

Library and Archives Canada Cataloguing in Publication

Parramore, Karin, 1964-, author
    Aromatherapy with essential oil diffusers : for everyday health & wellness /
Karin Parramore, LAc, CH.

Includes index.
ISBN 978-0-7788-0588-5 (softcover)

    1. Aromatherapy. 2. Essences and essential oils — Therapeutic use. I. Title.

RM666.A68P37 2017   615.3'219   C2017-905689-1

Index